The Encyclopedia
of Nursing Care Quality
Volume III

Monitoring
and Evaluation
in Nursing

The Encyclopedia
of Nursing Care Quality

The Encyclopedia
of Nursing Care Quality
Volume III

Monitoring
and Evaluation
in Nursing

Edited by
Patricia Schroeder, MSN, RN
Quality Care Concepts
Thiensville, Wisconsin

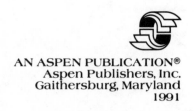

AN ASPEN PUBLICATION®
Aspen Publishers, Inc.
Gaithersburg, Maryland
1991

Library of Congress Cataloging-in-Publication Data

Monitoring and evaluation in nursing / edited by Patricia Schroeder.
p. cm. — (The Encyclopedia of nursing care quality : Vol. 3)
Includes bibliographical references and index.
ISBN: 0-8342-0217-4
1. Nursing audit. I. Schroeder, Patricia S. II. Series.
[DNLM: 1. Nursing Audit. WY 100.5 M744]
RT85.5.M66 1991
610.73 — dc20
DNLM/DLC
for Library of Congress
90-14564
CIP

Editorial Services: Ruth Bloom

Library of Congress Catalog Card Number: 90-14564
ISBN: 0-8342-0217-4
SERIES ISBN: 0-8342-0219-0

Printed in the United States of America

1 2 3 4 5

To my husband Steve and daughter Amy
for their love and encouragement

To my parents Irene and Walter
for their faith and guidance

To my family Jeanne, Charles, Michael, Elizabeth, and Timothy
for their friendship and support

Table of Contents

Contributors

Michael R. Bleich, MPH, RN, CNAA
Vice President for Nursing
Bryan Memorial Hospital
Lincoln, Nebraska
Healthcare Consultant
Quality Healthcare Resources, Inc.
Chicago, Illinois

Angeline Bushy, PhD, RN
Assistant Professor
College of Nursing Community Health
University of Utah
Salt Lake City, Utah

Marie J. Driever, PhD, RN
Assistant Director of Nursing
Quality Assurance/Research
Providence Medical Center
Portland, Oregon

Anne-Marie Duquette, RN, MS
President
Executive Nurse Consultants
Holliston, Massachusetts

Mary E. Barna Elrod, BSN, RN
Coordinator
Nursing Quality Assurance
University of Nebraska Medical Center
Omaha, Nebraska

Ann Libka Hendrich, MSN, RN
Clinical Research Nurse
Medical Research/Critical Care
Methodist Hospital of Indiana Inc.
Indianapolis, Indiana

Claire Meisenheimer, PhD, RN, CNAA
Associate Professor
University of Wisconsin
College of Nursing
Graduate Program
Oshkosh, Wisconsin

Jane A. Miller, RN, MSN, CPQA
Quality Assurance Project Specialist
Ambulatory Care Services Department
Methodist Hospital of Indiana, Inc.
Indianapolis, Indiana

Tari V. Miller, RN, MS
Former Assistant Administrator/Resident Care
Lakeland Nursing Home of Walworth County
Elkhorn, Wisconsin

Luc R. Pelletier, MSN, RN, CS
Regional Clinical Specialist
Psychiatric Institutes of America, Inc.
Long Beach, California
Former Director, Quality Management

Assistant Hospital Administrator
UCLA Neuropsychiatric Institute and
 Hospital
Assistant Clinical Professor
UCLA School of Nursing
Los Angeles, California

**Marilyn J. Rantz, RN, MSN,
 NHA**
Administrator
Lakeland Nursing Home of Walworth County
Elkhorn, Wisconsin

Paul A. Reichelt, PhD
Associate Professor
Department of Administrative Studies in
 Nursing
College of Nursing
University of Illinois at Chicago
Chicago, Illinois

Patricia Schroeder, MSN, RN
Nursing Quality Consultant
Quality Care Concepts
Thiensville, Wisconsin

Series Preface

Quality is being touted as the "make it or break it" issue of the decade—a concept that holds true in many aspects of American society. It has, however, become an urgent message in health care.

Quality has been brought to center stage for the nineties. Literature and experience tells us that quality is not only a concern of many—from governmental and accrediting agencies to special interest groups—but it also makes good business sense. The cost of good quality is less than the cost of poor quality. Quality enhances not only the receiver of care, but also the providers of care and services and the very state of the organization. It has been placed at the top of the agenda for organizations, administrators, practitioners, payers, and consumers alike. Quality in health care is being discussed, measured, and actually improved.

The Encyclopedia of Nursing Care Quality, a three volume series, contains descriptions of ongoing work to improve health care quality. Chapters written by noted experts in the field of nursing care quality take traditional nursing quality assurance activities and stretch them with applications of new approaches and refreshed enthusiasm. Recurring themes include the concepts of quality improvement, organizational culture, professional accountability, empowerment of those delivering the work of the organization, and collaboration for quality. It describes not just what is, but also what could, should, and will improve patient outcomes.

Volume I: Issues and Strategies in Nursing Care Quality takes a broad look at quality issues and programs in health care. Chapters include descriptions of state of the art programs to improve nursing care quality. Discussions of excellence in organizations, cost, automation, ethics, collaboration, program evaluation, and nursing QA coordinator roles are also contained in this valuable text.

Volume II: Approaches to Nursing Standards provides an overview of some of the most effective standards models used in today's health care settings. These models have unique features, and are described in relation to not only content and format, but also organizational systems and professional accountability. This text is unique in its ability to provide the reader with enough information to allow comparison and contrast between the approaches described. Other chapters discuss issues relevant to nursing standards including the importance of standards, validating standards, and legal issues in relation to standards. A description of the work of the American Nurses Association and the Nursing Organization Liaison Forum to develop national standards and guidelines is also contained in this volume.

Volume III: Monitoring and Evaluation in Nursing describes real world examples of the use of the ten step process in various specialty practice settings for nursing. "How to" discussions are followed by descriptions of unique features of monitoring and evaluating in different practice arenas such as medical-surgical units, mental health facilities, critical care, and long-term care. Ambulatory care and home care settings are also described. Other chapters discuss monitoring the use of the nursing process, using statistics in QA, clinical interpretation of data, and changing practice. This text provides the reader with many examples and thought provoking issues regarding the monitoring process.

This exciting set of books provides nurses with an overview of where we've been, where we are, and where we're going in the name of quality care. It is gratifying to see progress in a field that remained far too dormant for far too long. But perhaps more exhilarating is the clear message that nurses are making great strides in changing organizations for the wellbeing of patients, and improving the quality of health care for the American public.

Patricia Schroeder MSN, RN
Series Editor

Preface

"There is an ongoing quality assurance program designed to objectively and systematically monitor and evaluate the quality and appropriateness of patient care, pursue opportunities to improve patient care, and resolve identified problems." (Joint Commission, 1991)

Monitoring and evaluation of patient care have come to comprise the process used to measure the quality of care in health care organizations. As described by the Joint Commission on Accreditation of Healthcare Organizations, it is a way to identify those aspects of care most important to patient well-being, measure their important components, and make improvements based on the results. Given that the Joint Commission has articulated the expectation for monitoring and evaluation within its standards, and given that the Joint Commission is probably the single greatest influence on the structure and approach to quality assurance (QA) in this country, we in health care monitor and evaluate.

Literature from the Joint Commission describes monitoring and evaluation in a generic sense. The words used to describe the ten-step process are the same, irrespective of the clinical discipline or the setting under discussion. That makes sense because the overall process is the same. And yet differences in its application and ultimately its utility can be identified between specialty practice areas and clinical settings. Monitoring on a medical surgical unit is different from monitoring in ambulatory care. Monitoring critical care differs from monitoring in a mental health setting. But how? The unique features of monitoring the quality of nursing care from one setting to another have received little attention in professional literature.

Monitoring and Evaluation in Nursing describes the unique perspectives that play a role in carrying out QA activities in different specialty practice areas and in different practice settings. It is written by nurse experts who live with such QA programs and issues on a day-to-day basis. These nurses are professionals who not only understand the theory behind quality assurance, but also work hands-on in the practice field. My thanks to them for sharing their experience and expertise. This book is rich with examples of scopes of care and service, clinical indicators, and patient outcomes. It describes dilemmas and opportunities that present specific to the setting and its characteristics. Nurses who practice in a specific setting will be able to contrast their experience with that of these national authorities. Nurses who coordinate QA activities across several units will be able to identify issues that help them tailor their approaches and meet the needs of the various settings.

This book was created to provide clear descriptions of monitoring practice in different arenas. It is directly applicable to the clinical setting. It will provide you, the reader, with substance to move immediately in creating or improving your program.

Patricia Schroeder, MSN, RN
April 1991

REFERENCE

Joint Commission on Accreditation of Healthcare Organizations. (1991). *Accreditation Manual for Hospitals*. Chicago: Author.

1

Monitoring and Evaluation: An Introduction

Patricia Schroeder, MSN, RN, Nursing Quality Consultant, Quality Care Concepts, Thiensville, Wisconsin

All quality assurance (QA) or improvement programs involve the measurement of key indicators of quality. Irrespective of the quality philosophy espoused by a professional or an organization, some method of measurement must be carried out to determine attainment of standards or levels of practice, outcome, or performance. In health care settings, this measurement is currently called *monitoring and/ or evaluation*.

Although QA activities of some sort have been found in health care settings since the 1960s, the process of "monitoring practice" was only incorporated into the QA standards of the Joint Commission on Accreditation of Healthcare Organizations in 1984. Given that the Joint Commission has probably been the single greatest factor responsible for defining approaches to be taken to health care–related QA activities, this quickly became a national movement. Prior to that time, the focus of the Joint Commission's QA standards had evolved from chart audits to problem identification. The shift to ongoing, systematic monitoring was a significant advancement in the approach to measuring and improving quality.

Monitoring is defined as "the systematic and ongoing collection and organization of data related to the indicators of the quality and appropriateness of important aspects of care and the comparison of cumulative data with thresholds for evaluation related to each indicator" (Joint Commission, 1988, p. 148). Simply stated, monitoring is the measurement of small, but important, parts of care, practice, or staff performance. This measurement must be well planned, organized, and carried out using a sound approach. The resulting data must be reviewed at a reasonable time interval, as determined by members of the organization, and judgments made as to whether a problem exists. If problems are identified, either further and more extensive measurement is necessary, or some actions must be taken to resolve them.

Evaluation is defined as the "review and assessment of the quality and appropriateness of an important aspect of care" (Joint Commission, 1988, p. 147).

1

Evaluation is considered to be a more comprehensive study of a problematic aspect of care or practice. Rather than measuring a small part of that aspect of care or practice, a study is developed to take a closer look at the variables that have influenced the deficits and thereby better identify approaches to how the problem can be resolved.

Debate has raged for years over whether QA evaluation can be considered research. Many have suggested that evaluation as a process is on a continuum, with one end being simple problem evaluation and the other end sophisticated research. Movement on this continuum is based on the degree of scientific rigor employed in the process. Schmitt (1986) states that the differences between the research process and related processes such as clinical problem solving, program evaluation, and quality assurance are (1) the overall purpose of the activities and (2) the degree of rigor used in the collection and analysis of the data. Smeltzer and Hinshaw (1988) concur and further suggest that the major differences between research and QA studies are ''1) the purpose and 2) how the study results are utilized. The purpose of a quality assurance program is to assure the public that a system for evaluating and correcting nursing care problems is in place. The purpose of a research project is to provide information for administrative and clinical policy decisions as well as to add to the theoretical knowledge'' (pp. 38–39).

As health care professionals have gained experience in the process of monitoring and evaluation, several consistent premises can be identified as differentiating successful from unsuccessful approaches. Success in this instance is determined by the yielding of useful results that lead to improvements in care and practice. Success in nursing QA programs is also determined by the degree to which professional nurses feel empowered to implement changes that will result in quality improvements. Exhibit 1-1 lists those issues.

A PLANNED AND ORGANIZED APPROACH

In the mid-1980s, many struggled with the concept of monitoring. Approaches used were commonly fragmented, disorganized, and superficial. Many identified

---

Exhibit 1-1 Characteristics of Monitoring and Evaluation

Monitoring and evaluation must be

- based on a planned and organized approach
- based on valid standards of care and practice
- sufficiently rigorous to produce usable results
- carried out with meaningful staff nurse involvement
- used to improve care and practice

monitoring indicators only after the previous set of indicators was "finished." Rather than measuring the most essential indicators of care, many simply sought potentially quantifiable and accessible data. This often focused on what the nurse documented.

In 1987, the Joint Commission developed the ten-step process for monitoring and evaluation, which provided greater structure and guidance for health care. This process emphasizes that monitoring activities must be based on cogent advance planning; a clear perspective of one's client groups, services, and clinical activities; and an ongoing commitment to the collection and use of clinical data for quality improvement. Monitoring and evaluation cannot be successful if carried out on a whim or without clear direction. They must follow a sound plan that addresses both how the process and program will be conducted and what will be measured.

VALID STANDARDS OF CARE AND PRACTICE

Standards define one's vision of quality care. They speak to the professional's use of the nursing process to deliver care. They articulate values about important aspects of care and practice. And they incorporate the scientific base of the nursing profession into the process of defining diagnostic categories, interventions, and expected outcomes. Monitoring programs measure important components of practice in an attempt to identify opportunities to improve care. The concepts of standards and monitoring are intimately related. Yet, in many clinical settings, distinctly different structures have been created to develop and use standards and monitoring. While these concepts may have no relationship or integration in their application, the care delivered to patients in those settings must ultimately fit with both.

Standards commonly define projected patient goals and the nurse's approach to achieving them—outcomes and process. Monitoring programs too often focus on tasks, procedures, or aspects of documentation—process alone. An increasing emphasis on outcome measurement has been encouraged from many directions, including the Joint Commission, insurers who pay the costs of health care, the government, and consumers. Successful monitoring programs must integrate process and outcome measures of quality. They must also incorporate the essence of the care of the professional nurse. What are the most vital things nurses do in the delivery of professional nursing care? What are the essential outcomes patients must achieve? What differentiates professional nursing care from custodial care? "[O]ur systems invariably measure 'the wrong stuff.' We know how to measure costs—using models whose assumptions were created decades ago for a much different world. [Characteristics of true quality] are virtually absent from most measurement systems" (Peters, 1987, p. 583). As nurses, we must be sure that our standards define "the right stuff" and that our practice and ultimately its measurement are based on these standards.

SUFFICIENT RIGOR TO PRODUCE USABLE RESULTS

Hinshaw and Smeltzer (1987) describe the importance of time and resources in the conduct of research. "Research requires a great deal of time. The scientific inquiry process as a careful, systematic consideration of numerous details in the multiple phases of planning, implementation, analysis, and interpretation of data requires a long term commitment and understanding of a need for attention to such detail" (p. 22). Research, they say, is intended to generate new knowledge and to provide generalizable theory for the profession—and may identify causal links between variables.

In contrast, QA evaluation is intended to measure and improve the care provided in a given clinical agency to a specific population by scientific practitioners. Clinical evaluation for the purpose of quality improvement must be carried out in a manner that is realistic in regard to time, capability, and resources, and yet is sufficiently rigorous to allow confidence in the resulting data. This creates many dilemmas: How good is good enough? Are the data sufficiently solid to initiate organizational change in response?

MEANINGFUL STAFF NURSE INVOLVEMENT

Much has been written about the value of involving the bedside practitioners in the conduct of quality assurance. Deurr and Staats (1988) suggest that staff nurses are more readily able to identify clinical problems and that these nurses' "commitment is increased when involved in the control of what is to be monitored" (p. 14). Beyerman (1987) states that involving staff nurses is efficient because of the nurses' ability (1) to monitor functions on the unit while caring for patients and (2) to remedy deficiencies and create change as a result of a pre-established relationship with others on the unit and an understanding of unit values. Kraft, Neubauer, and LeSage (1987) state that monitoring by professional nurses experienced in the practice setting is essential because of the nurses' professional decision-making abilities. Schroeder (1988, 1990) and Formella and Schroeder (1984) have described many benefits of staff nurse involvement in quality measurement and improvement, as well as many benefits to quality care as a result of such involvement.

While the literature abounds with such comments, nurses in practice settings are increasingly stretched with greater patient needs and fewer resources with which to meet them. Furthermore, nurses involved in QA activities too often simply collect data. Examples of successful quality improvement programs in industries outside of health care reinforce the belief that those delivering health care must be involved in the measurement and improvement of quality. Monitoring and evaluation must be built into the roles of and expectations for all practitioners. Quality improvement philosophy has also been integrated into the Agenda for Change of the Joint Commission, further supporting the importance of staff involvement.

Staff nurses' most valuable role in monitoring is not collecting data, but using such data to improve care and practice. Only the careful analysis of monitoring data and the strategic implementation of change will result in benefits to the patient, the staff, and the organization. Monitoring and evaluation must incorporate the values, spirit, and perspectives of the staff to achieve their greatest potential.

IMPROVED CARE AND PRACTICE

"Measurement is too often equated with how many pounds of numerical indicators the senior manager receives weekly. There is little feel for the data at any level. Line—especially front line—involvement in its use or formulation is limited" (Peters, 1987, p. 583). While Peters is not speaking specifically of health care settings, the parallels can be easily drawn. All too often, health care practitioners function as if QA activities are completed with the phase of data collection. The value of monitoring and evaluation is not simply in their conduct or in the development of impressive reports. They are of value only if they have assured or are used to improve quality and/or practice.

Current emphasis on quality improvement, rather than quality assurance, fits with this perspective. Monitoring is seen not as a way to find fault, but instead as a strategy to find opportunities to improve. Its ultimate purpose is to create positive change. Such change not only benefits patients and the organization, but also circularly serves to reinvest nurses in the benefits of participation in the quality program.

The pursuit of quality in health care has had a strange evolution. While committed to providing the American public with quality care, health care professionals have structured approaches in the pursuit of quality that primarily meet the expectations of the Joint Commission. Such approaches have yielded mixed results in terms of actual benefits to care. Programs established to monitor and evaluate have stemmed from such beginnings, but have demonstrated potential for achieving both goals: improving care and meeting accrediting expectations. To achieve the greatest good, monitoring and evaluation must be carried out strategically, incorporating a dynamic structure, using an effective process, and pursuing valued outcomes.

REFERENCES

Beyerman, K. (1987). Developing a unit-based nursing quality assurance program: From concept to practice. *Journal of Nursing Quality Assurance, 2*, 1–11.

Deurr, B., & Staats, K. (1988). Quality assurance program evaluation: A view from the unit base. *Journal of Nursing Quality Assurance, 2*(4), 13–16.

Formella, N., & Schroeder, P. (1984). The unit-based system. In P. Schroeder and R. Maibusch (Eds.), *Nursing quality assurance: A unit-based approach* (pp. 29–49). Gaithersburg, MD: Aspen Publishers.

Hinshaw, A.S., & Smeltzer, C. (1987). Research challenges and programs for practice settings. *Journal of Nursing Administration, 17*(7,8), 20–26.

Joint Commission on Accreditation of Healthcare Organizations. (1988). *Guide to quality assurance.* Chicago: Author.

Kraft, M.R., Neubauer, J.A., & LeSage, J. (1987). Quality monitoring in long term care. *Journal of Nursing Quality Assurance, 2*(1), 39–48.

Peters, T. (1987). Thriving on chaos. Handbook for a management revolution. New York: Harper & Row.

Schmitt, M.H. (1986). The research process versus related processes. *Oncology Nursing Forum, 13*(4), 125–26, 131.

Schroeder, P. (1988). UBQA: A catalyst for professional development. In S.E. Pinkerton and P. Schroeder (Eds.), *Commitment to excellence: Developing a professional nursing staff* (pp. 29–32). Gaithersburg, MD: Aspen Publishers.

Schroeder, P. (1990). From the editor—Unit-based nursing quality assurance. *Journal of Nursing Quality Assurance, 4*(2), vii–viii.

Smeltzer, C., & Hinshaw, A.S. (1988). Research: Clinical integration for excellent patient care. *Nursing Management, 19*(1), 38–41.

2

Approaches to Monitoring Practice: Getting Started

Anne-Marie Duquette, RN, MS, President, Executive Nurse Consultants, *Holliston, Massachusetts*

NURSING QUALITY ASSURANCE

Monitoring practice is a process. The term *process* is used here to mean that monitoring practice can be approached as a progressive course of action, designed and implemented step by step. Nurses are familiar with another step-by-step process called the *nursing process*. The nursing process contains the steps of data gathering, assessment, planning, intervention, and evaluation (Fuerst, Wolff, & Weitzel, 1974, p. 52), whether practiced in a hospital setting, a home setting, a psychiatric center, or a long-term care facility. Similarly, the quality assurance (QA) process includes the same steps, regardless of the practice environment. No doubt clinical practice is very different in each setting, but the steps in the nursing process or the steps in the QA process remain the same in every environment.

HISTORICAL COMMITMENT TO QUALITY ASSURANCE

Throughout history, nurses have demonstrated their commitment to evaluating clinical practice patterns and identifying opportunities to improve care. During the Crimean War, Florence Nightingale reduced the mortality rate of soldiers from 42 percent to 2 percent by introducing standards of infection control and then comparing the care provided with the standards (Dock, 1925, p. 121).

During the 1950s, 1960s, and 1970s, process audits were introduced in an attempt to measure the quality of care provided by nurses. Examples of early audit tools include the Phaneuf Audit (Phaneuf, 1976), the Slater Scale (Wandelt & Stewart, 1975), the Quality Patient Care Scale (Qual PACs) (Wandelt & Ager, 1974), and the Rush Medicus Nursing Process Methodology (Jelinek et al., 1975). Each of the audits contained multiple criteria that gave nurses an opportunity to inspect and examine the process of providing care to patients.

Indeed, audit tools allowed for a comprehensive review of the process of providing care. Many, however, were very time consuming to use and lacked the flexibility necessary for users to select pertinent clinical criteria.

Faced with cost containment, shortages of health care workers, and reduced resources, nurses in the 1980s and 1990s look to QA activities to provide information essential in preserving needed services and personnel. Nurses are actively engaged in designing models and methods of monitoring practice that will allow for the evaluation of nursing care, and substantiate compliance with established standards of patient care.

QUALITY MONITORING SYSTEM REQUIREMENTS

When an architect begins designing a new building, certain building requirements must be considered and included in every building, regardless of the model. As nurses start monitoring practice ("doing QA"), certain requirements must be considered and included in every monitoring program.

First, QA monitoring must be planned. A written plan should describe how the monitoring process will be completed. The necessary components of a QA plan are discussed later in this chapter.

Next, the monitoring process must include every department or unit within the division of nursing. In an organization with 20 or 30 different specialties of nursing, all 20 or 30 units (i.e., psychiatry, medical nursing, surgical nursing, emergency services, endoscopy, radiology, clinics, operating room, etc.) must be involved in the process.

The process must be orderly. What was promised in the QA plan must be completed accurately and on time. Any variations from the plan must be explained in detail.

Monitoring, "the systematic collection and organization of data related to indicators of care" (Joint Commission, 1988, p. 148), must be ongoing. Once certain elements are selected for surveillance, these same elements are measured routinely in order to evaluate performance over a period of time. Quality assurance monitoring is a strategy for validating the consistency of compliance with clinical standards of practice.

The quality monitoring process must assure not only the quality of care, but also the appropriateness of care. Quality relates to the conformance to or variation from pre-established criteria, standards, policies, or procedures. Appropriateness refers to the fact that the standard being employed is relevant to the patient's condition. For example, nurses were monitoring compliance with a procedure for maintenance of skin integrity. The monitoring activity revealed that in 40 cases, the nurses adhered to the procedure 100 percent of the time. (Conformance with a pre-established procedure, quality). But in three cases, the patient's condition did not warrant the treatment. In these instances, the procedure standard was met, but the treatment was not appropriate. Monitoring activity must include both the quality of care and the appropriateness of care.

Finally, when opportunities to improve care are identified, nurses are required to take actions to improve care. The steps involved in planning and implementing corrective actions plans are discussed later in this chapter.

SELECTING A NURSING QA MODEL

As discussed throughout *The Encyclopedia of Nursing Care Quality*, there are many models of nursing QA programs. Many more models and approaches must still be developed as nurses attempt to realistically define, measure, and evaluate the quality to appropriateness of nursing care. In selecting or developing a model, nurses might take the following issues into consideration:

- Select or develop a structure that fits with the organizational structure and the style of management practiced in the organization.
- Decide on a format that makes the best use of the resources and manpower available.
- Keep the format simple and streamlined.
- Use a consistent model throughout the division of nursing.
- In a skilled nursing facility, use a consistency model throughout the facility.

THE JOINT COMMISSION'S TEN-STEP MONITORING AND EVALUATION PROCESS

In 1987, the Joint Commission on Accreditation of Healthcare Organizations published a ten-step process for the monitoring and evaluation of patient care. This process sets forth a step-by-step method for monitoring or measuring parts of professional practice in organizations. "The JCAHO is the nation's largest healthcare accrediting body with nearly 8,300 healthcare organizations accredited" (Joint Commission, 1987). Health care organizations seeking Joint Commission accreditation are currently expected to address the ten steps in their QA programs.

The ten-step monitoring process can also be a helpful approach in facilities and agencies that are not accredited by the Joint Commission. Many agencies and facilities that receive Medicare or Medicaid reimbursement are required to conduct QA activities. For example, after October 1, 1990, long-term care facilities are expected to have QA committees that meet at least quarterly to identify issues, develop corrective action plans, and correct identified problems, as required by the Omnibus Reconciliation Act of 1987 (P.L. 100-203), and stated in the *Federal Register* [54(21), February 2, 1989, p. 5,372]. The Joint Commission monitoring process includes the following steps:

1. Assign responsibility
2. Delineate the scope of care and service
3. Identify important aspects of care and service
4. Identify indicators related to the important aspects of care
5. Establish thresholds for evaluation
6. Collect and organize data
7. Evaluate care
8. Take action when opportunities for improvement or problems are identified
9. Assess the effectiveness of actions
10. Communicate relevant information to the organizationwide quality assurance committee (Joint Commission, 1989, p. 13)

Each of these steps will be discussed, with emphasis on practical implementation in health care settings.

Step 1: Assign Responsibility

According to the Joint Commission, "the nurse administrator is ultimately responsible for the implementation of a quality assurance program" (Joint Commission, 1990, p. 134). Completing step one of the Joint Commission's ten-step process requires writing a statement that describes who is responsible for making certain that QA activities are carried out in the facility.

Assigning responsibility should not be confused with assuming responsibility. Writing a nurse administrator's name on a QA plan or creating a list of names of responsible nurses is a superficial activity. Assuming responsibility for creating the support systems necessary for effective QA program implementation requires ongoing active participation in the monitoring process. Quality assurance activities can be a valuable source of data for administrators. Quality assurance processes identify, reduce, and prevent errors. Mistakes in patient care can be very expensive for patients and organizations in terms of prolonged illness, lost reimbursement, and legal fees.

Quality assurance has benefits beyond the identification of errors. Nurses can be empowered to be accountable for the practice of excellent nursing care using QA monitoring as a tool for identifying opportunities to improve patient care.

A QA system can become a catalyst in the professional development of the nursing staff. Nurses involved in quality assurance are required to

- conduct insightful assessments of their areas of practice while researching and writing a scope of care
- demonstrate accountability as they determine aspects of patient care that are essential to their areas of expertise
- apply basic research techniques as data-gathering strategies are designed and conducted
- communicate with peers and colleagues in other disciplines as the results of QA activities are analyzed and reported throughout the organization

Step 2: Delineate the Scope of Care and Service

Scope of care refers to the range of services provided to patients by a unit or department. "To delineate the scope of care for a given department personnel should ask themselves, 'What is done in the department?'" (Joint Commission, 1988, p. 52). This question is answered by preparing an inventory, including

- types of patients served
- conditions and diagnoses treated
- treatments or activities performed
- types of practitioners providing care
- sites where care is provided
- times when care is provided (Joint Commission, 1988, p. 52)

There are two ways to address the scope of care. The first approach is to take an organizational perspective. This is particularly valuable for organizations that serve a population of patients who are very similar and for facilities that have selected a centralized strategy for QA monitoring. For example, in a long-term care facility, it may be possible to state the following as a scope of care:

Scope of Care: ABC Nursing Home is a 75-bed, level-skilled nursing facility. Our residents range in age from 57 years old to 102 years old. Residents are admitted with multisystem health care problems. The problems range from acute and organic impairments to psychosocial deficits. Services rendered to residents include nursing, medical, psychiatric, social, spiritual, rehabilitative, and restorative activities to provide chronic short- and long-term care. Our staff is responsible for patient hygiene, patient comfort and safety, interventions to maintain mobility and nutritional well-being, patient and family education and counseling, and patient advocacy. Our services are provided 24 hours a day by a dedicated interdisciplinary staff consisting of nurse practitioners, registered nurses, licensed practical nurses, nurse's aides, social workers, physical therapists, dieticians, occupational/recreational therapists, and a physician advisor.

The second approach to delineating the scope of care would apply to a facility serving a diverse population. The scope of care might be more useful when each unit or special service describes its unique scope of care.

Scope of Care: Postpartum unit—The purpose of the unit is to provide physical, emotional, and educational support for mothers immediately after the birth of a baby.

What types of patients are served? Unit Postpartum cares for mothers and infants who are intermediate to low risk. All high-risk mothers are transferred to a local tertiary care center. In the event that a high-risk infant is born in our hospital, the neonatal intensive care team from the tertiary care center is contacted, and the team transports the infant to the tertiary care center.

List the conditions and diagnoses treated. The conditions and diagnoses treated on our unit are normal postpartum care and newborn care.

List the treatments or activities performed. Our treatments and activities center around the comfort and education of our mothers and the care and feeding of our newborns. Our services include family-centered education and counseling, promotion of patient safety, management of complications associated with childbirth, and patient referral.

State the practitioners providing care. Our unit employs an inter-disciplinary approach to the care of mothers and infants. Services are provided by physicians, nurses, aides, social workers, and dieticians.

Identify the site where care is provided. Unit Postpartum is a 37-bed unit located on the fourth floor of building B in City Hospital.

State the times when care is provided. Unit Postpartum offers care 24 hours a day. The average length of stay is two days for a vaginal delivery and three days for a Caesarean delivery. Home care services are offered to all patients.

Step 3: Identify Important Aspects of Care and Service

Important aspects of nursing care can best be described as some of the fundamental contributions made by nurses while caring for patients. They are the most significant or essential categories of care practiced in a given setting. There is no prescribed list of important aspects of care that every organization must monitor. Rather, selecting important aspects of care is a contemplative step that must be completed by informed practitioners in every unit, department, or facility. Aspects of care are broad categories of professional nursing behavior or patient attributes; among the more important are

- patient assessment
- care planning
- patient education
- discharge planning
- referral
- patient transfer
- maintenance of skin integrity
- pain management
- maintenance of mobility
- maintenance of nutritional balance
- counseling
- patient/family satisfaction
- administration of medications
- prevention of patient injury
- prevention of patient falls
- restraint of patients
- prevention of infections

In a centralized approach to monitoring nursing practice, aspects of care can be listed for the entire nursing division and possibly included in the nursing QA program plan, discussed later in this chapter.

When using a unit-based approach, each unit identifies its unique aspects of care. Nurses in the emergency room, for example, may select one aspect of care related to patient education regarding follow-up procedures. On a postpartum unit, the nursing staff may instead be very concerned with patient education about breastfeeding. Unit-based quality assurance allows nurses to identify the unique needs of patients and the specific priorities of their caregivers. In addition, empowering nurses to identify unit-specific aspects of care offers an opportunity to develop the clinical accountability of the nursing staff.

Step 4: Identify Indicators Related to the Important Aspects of Care

"From the perspective of JCAHO, a clinical indicator is a quantitative measure that can be used as a guide to monitor and evaluate the quality of important patient care and support service activities" (Characteristics, 1989, p. 330). For example, the incidence of skin breakdown in a long-term care facility could be considered a measurable outcome of the effectiveness of nursing interventions to maintain skin integrity. Using the QA nomenclature, the important aspect of care would be maintenance of skin integrity. The measurable indicator would be the number of cases of skin breakdown.

Some indicators are broad and are based on the achievement of several more specific measures. These specific measures, often subsumed within the indicator, may be called *subindicators, criteria,* or *data elements.*

Indicators are currently considered as being of two general types, sentinel event and rate-based. "A sentinel event indicator measures serious, undesirable, and often avoidable process or outcomes" (Characteristics, 1989, p. 332). For example, when a patient falls and breaks a hip, this would be considered a sentinel event. Although sentinel events are usually low in number and may not be identified as a trend or pattern over time, the single event is of such a serious nature that it triggers an opportunity to improve care. A rate-based indicator measures patient care events over time. Thresholds are set for rate-based indicators. Therefore, investigations of rate-based indicators are usually triggered when the predetermined threshold for that indicator is exceeded. For example, "7.1% of residents in skilled nursing facilities nationally have one or more decubitus ulcers" (Health Care Financing Administration, 1988). Seven percent could be set as the threshold for the indicator "incidence of skin breakdown in a skilled nursing facility"; such an indicator would be described as a rate-based indicator.

Indicators also differ according to the type of event they usually measure: structure, process, or outcome. "Structure indicators measure elements that facilitate care, such as resources, equipment, or numbers and qualifications of staff" (Joint Commission, 1989, p. 18). For example: "One flotation mattress will be kept in stock on every nursing unit." Having a flotation mattress in stock on each unit may be used as a structural indicator regarding availability of equipment necessary to maintain patients' skin integrity.

"Processes are those functions carried out by practitioners, such as assessment, treatment, planning, and so forth" (Joint Commission, 1989, p. 18). "Process indicators generally seek to measure discrete steps in the patient care process that are important" (Characteristics, 1989, p. 332). An example of a process indicator used in monitoring and evaluating nursing practice with regard to the maintenance of skin integrity could be written as follows: "Within four hours of admission, the patient's skin condition will be assessed."

The indicator "numbers of cases of skin breakdown" would be considered an outcome indicator. "Outcomes include complications, adverse events, and results of treatment" (Joint Commission, 1989, p. 18). "An outcome indicator measures what happens (or does not happen) to patients after something is done (or not done) to them" (Characteristics, 1989, p. 332). Since 1987, when the Joint Commission began an Agenda for Change, a great deal of emphasis has been placed on outcome monitoring. However, a comprehensive QA program usually includes all three types of indicators.

Regardless of the format, structure, process, or outcome, indicators should "possess certain attributes that together determine their utility as measures of care" (Characteristics, 1989, p. 333).

- Indicators must be valid. "Validity is the degree to which the indicator accomplishes its purpose—the identification of situations in which the quality of care and services should be improved" (Characteristics, 1989, p. 333). The state of the art in nursing quality assurance calls for reliance on face validity, rather than scientific validity. Face validity means that relationships that make sense to clinically competent nurses are measured. Scientific validity is based on documented research findings. As indicator development is a new technology, documented research material is not readily available. An indicator that measures the numbers of cases of skin breakdown is an excellent example of what might be considered a valid measurement within quality assurance circles.
- Indicators must be reliable. "Reliability is the ability of an instrument to obtain consistent results," (Treece & Treece, 1982, p. 119). If the unit or department monitors maintenance of skin integrity every month, the data should suggest a consistent pattern of results. Naturally, if an opportunity exists to improve care, the incidence may be higher during months in which problems exist.
- Indicators must be specific and measure only one variable at any one time. For example, an indicator that asks if a patient could state the time and dose of his or her discharge medications would be difficult to measure because two variables are stated, time and dose. Time could be one indicator, and dose could be a second indicator.
- Indicators must be sensitive and capture all cases of care in which quality of care issues exist. For example, "incidence of skin breakdown" captures all cases of skin breakdown and, therefore, all cases in which a quality of care issue could potentially exist.

Nurses concerned about the accuracy and legitimacy of their information must give careful consideration to the formulation of nursing care indicators. Consider the following examples:

Aspect of Care: Patient Education Regarding Self-Administration of Medication
Indicators:
- Each patient is able to
  1. identify his or her medication by sight
  2. state two potential side effects of his or her medication

Aspect of Care: Discharge Planning
Indicators:
- Each patient is able to describe what he or she is expected to do upon discharge with regard to
  1. activity level
  2. signs and symptoms that require a call to the doctor
  3. dietary restrictions
  4. names of medication prescribed

Aspect of Care: Maintenance of Skin Integrity
Indicator:
- Number of cases of skin breakdown that occur after admission

Aspect of Care: Patient/Family Satisfaction
Indicators:
- Patient/family would return for care if needed.
- Patient/family would refer people they know to the organization.

If indicators of care and aspects of care were parts of a book, an aspect of care would be the chapter title, and the indicators of care would be the subtitles throughout the chapter. A combination of aspects of care and indicators make up a table of contents. In a nursing service, a combination of aspects of care and indicators creates a profile of the quality of care provided. One aspect of care and one indicator must be viewed as only one portion of a chapter and, therefore, a very limited measure of the quality of care. Monitoring programs are intended to provide a survey of the quality of care, not detailed accounts of the activities of each caregiver and the experiences of every patient.

Step 5: Establish Thresholds for Evaluation

Thresholds are accepted levels of compliance with any indicators being measured. ''Thresholds for evaluation are the level or point at which intensive evaluation is triggered'' (Joint Commission, 1988, p. 53). Nurses must use clinical judgment to set thresholds.

A threshold can be viewed as a stimulus for action. Consider the following example in which nurses have determined that patients should be able to state two potential side effects of discharge medications 95 percent of the time. The results of cumulative data that were collected show that patients are able to state two potential side effects of discharge medications 75 percent of the time. The threshold, the percentage the nurses stated as the minimal level of acceptance, was not met. When a threshold is not met, all the data should be thoroughly analyzed to identify any opportunity that exists to improve patient care.

Following are important points to consider in setting thresholds:

- Thresholds are set for each indicator.
- Thresholds are most often set using the clinical judgment and experience of the nurses providing care.
- Nursing performance will be measured against the thresholds.
- Thresholds represent minimum levels of acceptable performance.
- Thresholds are usually set to reflect a high level of compliance because most indicators selected for monitoring are essential ingredients in patient care.
- Thresholds can reflect the presence of events (100 percent) or the absence of events (0 percent) or points in between.

Step 6: Collect and Organize Data

Methods

Once indicators have been identified, a method of collecting data about the indicators must be selected. Among the many methods of data collection are interviewing patients, interviewing families, distributing questionnaires, reviewing charts, making direct observations, and sharing information already being collected and reported on by other disciplines within the organization. Selecting a data collection method is an important step in the quality assurance process; but QA data collection techniques are not usually subjected to the ''scientific'' tests required for data collection tools intended for research purposes.

Interviewing. Each method of data collection has advantages and disadvantages. Interviewing patients and/or family members provides an excellent opportunity for patients and family members to express their perception of their caregivers. Conducting patient interviews, however, is very time consuming. Some patients may be hesitant or too sick to consent to an interview. Interviewers must avoid asking questions that would put patients or families in a vulnerable position, such as "Are the nurses providing good care?"

Distributing Questionnaires. A skillfully designed questionnaire is a great source of data, the key words being "skillfully designed." Each item on a questionnaire must be concisely and precisely worded to obtain reliable results. Questionnaires ought to be tested with small groups before soliciting information from an entire population of patients, family members, or staff nurses. Keep questionnaires brief; five to eight statements can provide ample information for quality monitoring. When writing questions, keep the reading level low, and avoid using health care terminology or jargon.

Reviewing Charts. Two types of chart review are worthy of note: concurrent chart review and retrospective chart review. With concurrent chart review, the documentation is examined while the patient is still receiving service. A retrospective chart review is conducted after a case is closed or after the client is discharged. Concurrent chart review has been regarded favorably in recent years, with the major concern being the importance of improving care while the patient is still receiving service. Looking at patients' records after discharge may highlight missed opportunities. Nevertheless, retrospective chart review may be the method of choice if nurses are monitoring, for example, their performance during the discharge process.

Making Direct Observations. To use observation as an effective data collection method, observers must be trained and be able to consider the effect that they might have on clinicians. Research has shown that the very fact that people are observing can change performance. Observation is valuable, however, when the data would not be completely reported or recorded elsewhere—for example, "the patient demonstrates correct self-injection of insulin."

Sharing Information. Great stores of data are available throughout an organization without instituting additional data collection methods. Since every department is required to conduct QA monitoring, the best place to start would be to find out about the data being collected and used by the following departments: infection control, medical staff, risk management, dietary, laboratory, pharmacy, safety/equipment, utilization review, nursing education, respiratory, physical therapy, occupational therapy, rehabilitation services, and social services. Members of these departments could already be collecting data that reflect the performance of both their own department and nursing. Use of such data can, at times, simplify data collection and provide valuable opportunities for interdepartmental collaboration for quality.

Sample Size

How much monitoring should be conducted by nurses on a monthly basis? There is no exact formula for determining how many cases to monitor. Some reviewers suggest examining five percent of all applicable cases. However, five percent of 40,000 cases would be unmanageable and totally unnecessary. For the most part, 20 cases reviewed each month for each indicator should result in sufficient information for analysis. In some cases, such as medication errors, the nurses would always review 100 percent of the cases that occurred.

Duration of Surveillance

In the past, many nurses were familiar with a process of review called an *audit* or a *problem-focused study*. This involved a one-time-only look at a clinical issue. Using the current terminology, *ongoing monitoring* refers specifically to collecting information about the same indicators every month or at routinely scheduled intervals. However, if nursing performance is found month after month to meet thresholds 100 percent of the time, competent clinicians will need to make a decision about how long to monitor indicators where there is an established pattern of 100 percent compliance with predetermined thresholds. Again, there is no exact formula to use as a guide when stopping surveillance, but four to six months of 100 percent compliance with any given threshold is ample evidence that there may be no opportunity to improve care. When ongoing monitoring of that indicator is being stopped, a clear rationale for the action must be stated in a subsequent QA report. Opportunities for improvement can then be sought through the use of other indicators.

Step 7: Evaluate Care

When data gathering is completed in the process of planning patient care, nurses make assessments based on the findings. In the QA process as a whole, when data collection has been completed and summarized, a group of nurses makes an assessment of the quality of care.

During the evaluation process, several questions might be answered. Were the thresholds set for each indicator met? In instances in which the thresholds were met, reports would be filed, the monitoring process would continue, and no further action would be required. When thresholds are not met, the following issues come to mind:

- Was the threshold set too high?
- Are there acceptable exceptions to the indicator?
- Were the indicators measurable and appropriate?
- Was an opportunity to improve care identified?

The data must be looked at from a clinical viewpoint. Only practicing clinicians have the perspective necessary to analyze the data and determine their clinical meaning and impact.

Step 8: Take Action To Resolve Identified Problems

Nurses are action-oriented professionals. For many nurses, the greater portion of every day is spent on patient intervention. These actions and interventions conducted by nurses promote health and wellness for patients.

Converting nursing energy into the QA process requires formulating an action plan to address identified problems. For example, if patients being discharged cannot state two potential side effects of their medications, what can nurses do to help them better learn this necessary information? The QA action plan might include the following:

- reporting all findings to the nursing staff to raise their awareness of the problem
- collaborating with physicians to identify, as early as possible, medications to be taken by the patient after discharge
- working with pharmacists to develop medication information cards on commonly prescribed drugs
- developing a procedure for distributing and reviewing medication cards with patients at the time of discharge
- identifying or clarifying who is responsible for carrying out this teaching
- sharing the information with other members of the health care team so they can include it in their teaching as well
- establishing a medication "hot line" so patients can call pharmacists with questions after discharge

These are but a few suggestions. Creative clinicians could identify many more based on their intimate knowledge of the patient groups with whom they work and the systems within which they function. Keep in mind that actions will improve care only if they are based on an accurate analysis of the clinical problem. Clinical practitioners need to be as specific as possible when creating corrective action plans.

Step 9: Assess the Effectiveness of Actions

Continuous and sustained improvement in care requires constant surveillance by nurses of the interventions initiated to improve care. Consider the following analogy. A newly diagnosed diabetic patient who has just been taught a 1,500 ADA diet often needs ongoing support and supervision when making dietary selections during the early stages of recovery. Changing behavior, adapting to new ways of thinking, and developing new habits or systems of conducting daily life take time and patience. Nurses should not act surprised when initial attempts to correct longstanding habits or problems seem to fail. Just because a problem has been found and reported does not mean that it will be immediately corrected or eliminated.

Step 10: Communicate Relevant Information to the Organizationwide QA Committee

Nursing represents one group of players on an organizational team. Written and verbal messages about the results of QA activities must be shared with other disciplines throughout the facility. Most important, nursing QA activities should be integrated with hospitalwide QA activities. Thus, a mechanism should be in place so nursing can report its findings to the organizationwide QA committee(s). In addition, the governing board of the organization carries overall responsibility for the organization, and QA activities must ultimately be reported to and reviewed by that governing board.

The Joint Commission's ten-step monitoring and evaluation process discussed thus far might be considered an explanation of the ingredients for a QA monitoring process. However, it is also important to write a QA plan for nursing service, using these ingredients. Although a nursing QA plan is not currently required by regulatory agencies, such a plan serves as a blueprint for action and a guide for colleagues involved in the QA process.

WRITING A QA PROGRAM PLAN

Step 1: Purpose or Goal

In stating the purpose, the following question should be answered: What is the intention of the quality assurance program? An example of what could be stated is this: "The purpose of the quality assurance program or the goal of the quality assurance program for nursing service is to establish a planned and systematic process for the monitoring and evaluation of the quality and appropriateness of patient care and for resolving identified problems" (Joint Commission, 1989, p. 142).

Step 2: Objectives

Objectives should define what is to be accomplished by carrying out a QA plan. Some plans include both long-term and short-term objectives. Long-term objectives act as a guide to the overall program; examples include

- evaluating compliance with the established standards of patient care
- monitoring patients' safety
- identifying problems
- developing strategies to resolve identified problems
- recognizing and improving the quality of nursing care provided to patients
- identifying nurses with performance problems

Short-term objectives reflect the emphasis for the next one or two years; examples include

- incorporating a two-hour class on quality assurance into orientation for new nurses
- conducting a half-day workshop for all QA representatives on how to write clinical indicators
- revising QA reporting tools
- researching and selecting a software package for sorting QA information and writing reports

Step 3: Describe Role Responsibilities

Although accountability for QA programs is the ultimate responsibility of a nurse administrator, in most organizations many nurses are involved in quality assurance. At this point in the plan, describe the roles and responsibilities of every member of the QA team. For example:

- *QA coordinator:* acts as a resource to staff nurses on QA issues; collates a quarterly summary of materials sent from all nursing areas; may be directly responsible for collecting data and creating quarterly reports, if the facility has a centralized QA program; creates and distributes the agenda for nursing QA meetings
- *Staff nurse:* identifies quality concerns on the unit or throughout the facility; helps collect data; participates in analysis of QA data; suggests corrective actions when indicated; performs corrective actions when appropriate

- *Nurse manager:* is responsible for the quality of care in his or her area of responsibility; can delegate QA responsibilities to experienced clinical nurses, support the staff nurses by providing time to carry out QA activities, and empower the staff nurses to act on their findings by allowing them to carry out corrective action plans
- *Unit representative or chairperson of the unit QA committee:* might coordinate QA activities on the unit; writes a report of these activities on a quarterly basis and sends it to the person who is coordinating quality assurance for the entire nursing service; holds monthly meetings with staff nurses or the unit QA committee to discuss QA activities and get feedback on results; keeps all QA written materials in good order on the nursing unit

Step 4: Describe a Structure

The structure should indicate the manner in which the work of quality assurance will be completed. State the particular model that has been chosen. If a unique model has been created at the facility, describe it, and include a diagram of the structure. Be sure to explain how this nursing department structure relates to the organizationwide QA program and how reports get to the governing board.

Step 5: Describe QA Committee Functions

The QA committee will oversee the process of monitoring nursing practice. Although some committee functions may be determined by the QA model selected, responsibilities that might be considered include

- meeting monthly
- conducting an annual evaluation of the QA program
- integrating nursing QA activities with organizationwide activities
- receiving and responding to reports about various QA activities
- providing ongoing education and training for nurses unfamiliar with the QA process

Step 6: State How Monitoring and Evaluation Will Be Conducted

For QA monitoring results to be useful, the information needs to be summarized. A convenient way to organize the QA reporting schedule is to collect data for three months (or one quarter) and then report the findings. As an example, in a program where monitoring started in January, data would be collected in January and February, and a report would be created at the end of March. Data would then be collected in April and May and reported in June, and so on. The schedule would look like this:

JAN	FEB	MAR	APR	MAY	JUN	JUL	AUG	SEP	OCT	NOV	DEC
C	C	R	C	C	R	C	C	R	C	C	R

C = Collect data   R = Report data

An alternative approach would be to stagger reports so that all units are not reporting at the same time. While these approaches reflect the "formal" time frames for reporting, any evidence of significant clinical problems must be followed up immediately.

Suggestions for Writing a Plan

Establishing the Reporting Format

When choosing a data-reporting format, be certain that other people will be able to understand what is being said. The report might include

- a list of all the QA activities that have been conducted within an identified time frame
- any trends identified and what is being done about them
- any problems that have been addressed
- follow-up action taken on any unresolved problems identified in previous reports

Preparing the Cover of the Plan

People spend a great deal of time writing a QA plan, but still forget to state some very important information on the cover—information that is easily forgotten one year later when it is time to conduct an annual review and, in some instances, long after the original author has left the organization. In order to promote continuity over time, consider including the following items on the cover:

- title of the program
- name of the organization
- address of the organization
- person(s) to whom the plan is being submitted

- person(s) who prepared the plan
- date the plan was submitted
- date the plan was approved

Organizing QA Materials

Keeping QA materials in good order is no small job! Following is a suggested order for QA materials which may be useful:

1. a copy of a current nursing service QA plan
2. in the case of a unit-based program, a unit-specific information sheet containing
   a. a list of nurses responsible for quality assurance on the unit
   b. a description of the scope of nursing care on the unit
   c. a list of important aspects of care
   d. a list of indicators for the important aspects of care that have been identified, with the thresholds that have been set
3. a space for correspondence; correspondence takes the subtle form of complaints from other disciplines, thank you notes from patients and families, reports from other departments (on, for example, infection rates, medication error rates, number of patient falls), memos from upper-level managers about specific performance issues, requests from the dieticians or laboratory staff, etc.
4. current summaries of all QA activities, with examples of monitoring tools
5. agendas and minutes from staff meetings in which the results of QA activities were discussed; be sure to state the staff's response to the results.
6. agendas and minutes from other QA committees with whom you collaborate
7. a list indicating all education provided based on QA activities and findings
8. a list that describes what the staff has learned from conducting QA reviews, highlighting any problems identified and any changes that have been made on the unit. The list might follow the format given below

Date	What We Learned	What We Changed	How It Worked

CONCLUSION

The implementation and ongoing administration of a nursing quality monitoring program must be efficient and effective. Major clinical decisions now and in the future will be based on the data obtained through quality monitoring efforts. The data, therefore, must be accurate and reflect the best interests of patients and nurses. The approaches selected when starting to monitor practice can determine the direction of nursing service and nursing practice within the organization. The keys to getting started are strategic planning, thorough preparation and education of the nursing staff, and carefully guided implementation.

REFERENCES

Dock, L.L. (1925). *A short history of nursing* (2nd ed.). New York: G.P. Putnam's Sons.

Fuerst, E.V., Wolff, L., & Weitzel, M.H. (1974). *Fundamentals of nursing* (5th ed.). Philadelphia: J.B. Lippincott.

Jelinek, R.C., Haussmann, R.K.D, Hegyvary, S.T., & Newman, S.F. (1975). *A methodology for monitoring quality nursing care.* Bethesda, MD: U.S. Department of Health, Education, and Welfare, U.S. Public Health Service, Health Resources Administration, Bureau of Health Manpower, Division of Nursing.

Joint Commission on Accreditation of Healthcare Organizations. (1987). *Facts about the Joint Commission, Overview of the Agenda for Change.* Chicago: Author.

Joint Commission on Accreditation of Healthcare Organizations. (1988). *Guide to quality assurance.* Chicago: Author.

Joint Commission on Accreditation of Healthcare Organizations. (1989). Characteristics of clinical indicators. *Quality Review Bulletin,* 330–339.

Joint Commission on Accreditation of Healthcare Organizations. (1989). *Update on nursing services monitoring and evaluation.* Chicago: Author.

Joint Commission on Accreditation of Healthcare Organizations. (1990). *Accreditation manual for hospitals.* Chicago: Author.

Phaneuf, M. (1976). *The nursing audit: Profile for excellence.* New York: Appleton-Century-Crofts.

Schroeder, P.S. (1991). *The Encyclopedia of Nursing Care Quality.* Gaithersburg, MD: Aspen Publishers.

Treece, E.W., & Treece, J.W., Jr. (1982). *Elements of research in nursing.* St. Louis: C.V. Mosby.

U.S. Department of Health and Human Services, Health Care Financing Administration. (1989, February 2). Medicare and Medicaid; Requirements for long term care facilities; Final rule with request for comments. *Federal Register, 54*(21), 5,359–5,373.

Wandelt, M.A., & Ager, J.W. (1974). *Quality patient care scale.* New York: Appleton-Century-Crofts.

Wandelt, M.A., & Stewart, D.S. (1975). *Slater nursing competencies rating scale.* New York: Appleton-Century-Crofts.

3

Quality Assurance: Challenges and Dilemmas in Acute Care Medical-Surgical Environments

Mary E. Barna Elrod, BSN, RN, Coordinator, Nursing Quality Assurance, University of Nebraska Medical Center, Omaha, Nebraska

Nursing care of medical-surgical (M-S) patients in acute care facilities has changed drastically over the past decade in response to such major influences as social trends, consumer demands, technological advances, and altered methods of financing health care. Gone are the days of the "general med-surg" patient. Today's patient presents a variety of new and different challenges within an evolving specialty area. Creative and innovative changes will be needed to respond to the needs of this patient population group—quality assurance (QA) being foremost among them.

This chapter presents an overview of the changing medical-surgical environment and describes real-world issues unique to monitoring nursing care and patient outcomes in an acute care facility. Opportunities for and constraints on QA program success specific to this practice setting are discussed. Examples of monitoring and evaluation methodologies developed by practitioners in medical-surgical areas are included.

ENVIRONMENTAL INFLUENCES AFFECTING MEDICAL-SURGICAL ENVIRONMENTS

Today's consumers of health care are more interested in and concerned about their involvement in decisions affecting their lives. They want to be active participants, not passive recipients, with regard to factors affecting their personal health and well-being. Consumers' growing interest in the health industry evolved from the impersonal technological emphasis of the 1950s and resulted in a growing mistrust of institutions (Naisbitt, 1982). People became more self-reliant as a result of this mistrust. Their changing demands and growing dissatisfaction with the health care industry have prompted that industry to become consumer driven and to strive to improve the quality of its services. Providers of health services can no longer create the services they want to deliver and expect the customer to consume them (Peterson, 1988).

As consumers developed greater expectations regarding health care, the federal government became more active in the financing of health care. As a result, regulations regarding the cost and quality of services were formulated in the 1960s (Bull, 1985). Health care does have a price, and this became evident over the next 20 years as inflation and the cost of health care continued to increase. Easterbrook (1987) reported the total U.S. health spending for 1985 was $425 billion. Something had to be done to control the escalating cost. What resulted were decreases in health care funding by public, private, and governmental agencies. This, in turn, caused the development of numerous strategies to manage the cost of health care. Examples include preadmission screening, second opinions for surgery, utilization review, prospective payment systems, diagnostic related groups, and health maintenance organizations. These financial constraints forced the health care industry to shift its focus from inpatient acute care to other, cheaper methods of care delivery, including outpatient surgical centers, ambulatory care, home care, and community care.

As a result of this decreased funding and increased emphasis on alternate care delivery methods, patients are hospitalized less frequently, have higher levels of acuity, require more complex and intense nursing care, and stay for shorter periods of time. In the past, these patients might have been admitted to an intensive care/ special care unit, but are now routinely seen in "general" M-S units.

Competition among hospitals for ailing bodies has dramatically increased in attempts to counter decreasing total patient days. Using strategic planning and marketing approaches, facilities in a given community try to outdo each other by offering special services or treatments of high quality by competent staff at a competitive rate. Examples include organ and tissue transplants, medical and surgical oncology programs, gerontological services, dysrhythmia monitoring, acute/chronic cardiopulmonary services, and autoimmune or infectious disease treatment. Since most facilities cannot afford special units for each type of service they capitalize on, their patients are most likely to be hospitalized on M-S units. Thus, the diagnostic population mix on any given M-S unit can be extremely diverse, with each one requiring unique, complex, and intense care. The technological advances developed to monitor, test, and treat the multiple physical parameters of this varied population mix add to the complexity of knowledge and ethical thinking needed by the nurses to practice M-S nursing.

Poteet and Hodges (1987) identified some important major social trends that undoubtedly will also influence the type of patient ultimately admitted to M-S units. Among them are the growing percentage of people over age 65, the rapid expansion of minority and immigrant populations, increasing poverty, and the fear of health care rationing due to shrinking health dollars. If these trends continue, one can expect that older patients will occupy the majority of acute care beds, women (if they continue to live longer than men) will be the dominant sex seen, a wide variety of cultural groups will be represented, and ethical and moral dilemmas will proliferate due to allocation of scarce resources. An examination of each of these points may emphasize the realities of these predictions.

America has not traditionally valued its older citizen, and as a result, the health industry has not given enough attention to the diagnosis, treatment, or prevention of health problems for this age group. Currently, the number of people over 65 years old is growing at approximately twice the rate of the general population. By the year 2000 they will represent over 13 percent of the population (Poteet & Hodges, 1987).

Acute care facilities are cognizant of the increasing numbers of elderly among their population as they struggle to maintain fiscal viability within federally mandated reimbursement guidelines. Some are responding by physically locating people aged 65 and over in ''special'' acute care geriatric units or centers within their facilities. Research is not yet available to validate the financial impact or care outcomes for these patients. However, it is unrealistic to believe that clustering older patients in a particular location is either desirable or feasible for all acute care facilities. Thus, the elderly will continue to be hospitalized in increasing numbers on M-S units.

Besides increases in the number of elderly, other shifts in the patient population of M-S units are anticipated. Poteet and Hodges (1987) emphasize that the Hispanic population will outnumber the black population by 1990, making Hispanics the largest minority sector in America. Because immigrants to America come from all over the world, our cultural diversity has increased. People of different minorities, cultures, and ethnic backgrounds will be seen with increasing frequency as citizens of our country and as patients in our acute care M-S beds. Greater understanding of the uniqueness, differences, concerns, and problems of these various groups of Americans will be needed. Medical-surgical nurses will be challenged by such things as language barriers, dietary preferences, different family dynamics, religious preferences, varied educational backgrounds, and social-cultural norms unique to each group.

The growing number of this nation's poor will certainly have an impact on altering the acute care M-S environment: There may be very few or an overabundance of poor patients admitted to them. The bottom line is money. It takes money to run a business, and the health care industry does not benefit financially from caring for the poor. Besides having no money, the poor lack private insurance. Easterbrook (1987) reports that in 1982 there were 37 million people under the age of 65 who had no insurance. It is suspected that this number is greater today. Many of the poor may not be eligible for Medicaid coverage. Although Medicaid is a federal program, it is administered by the states. It is, therefore, without uniform federal standards, and the quality of the individual programs can vary greatly from state to state.

Poor patients without any insurance or those unable to make a down payment may not even be admitted to a growing number of hospitals. Those seen in an emergency department may be quickly transferred to the nearest city or county hospital that receives tax support. Morally, this should not be a concern if the quality of care at public facilities is equal to care given at private facilities, as demonstrated by patient outcomes and adherence to acceptable standards of practice. It is, however, morally wrong when two standards of care—one for those who can pay and one for those who cannot—are evident. As the health dollar continues to shrink, this separation will become more evident unless major revisions in the system are made.

Nurses caring for an overabundance of poor patients in their M-S units will continue to do the best they can to provide for a population that cannot compete equally with the middle or the upper income class. The poor may be sicker due to delays in seeking prompt medical attention, inadequate housing, poor dietary habits, and lack of proper education. Personal, social, community, and federal resources do not allow these nurses to do much more. Nurses caring for an occasional poor patient among their cases may have more resources to tap into to temporarily intervene in the poor patient's behalf. Examples of financial relief efforts demonstrated by nurses include initiating fund-raising drives to help pay for the cost of an operation or hospitalization, collecting donations of food and clothing from staff and the community, and providing nursing care in a less expensive way (e.g., very early discharge, nonuse of prepackaged treatment/procedure kits). Helping an occasional poor person seen on M-S units is certainly admirable, but will become extremely difficult if the number of the poor in M-S beds increases.

The plight of the poor demonstrates an example of the emerging ethical and moral dilemmas that health care rationing, under the guise of resource allocation, presents for society to ponder. Questions that need to be addressed in order to help identify and ultimately resolve ethical concerns include these: Is access to health care a "right" guaranteed by the Constitution? What is an equitable way to provide health care without regard to socioeconomic status, race, or ethnic origin? Should health dollars and services be provided where they can accomplish the greatest good for the most people? Does American society have any special health obligations to its elderly or poor? Is transferring an indigent person for other than medical reasons acceptable? Nurses in M-S units, as advocates for patients, will increasingly be challenged to find ways through QA activities to assure and demonstrate that standards of care are equally applied to all patient groups.

AN EMERGING SPECIALTY AREA

Nurse educators and administrators of the past usually advised a new graduate to get some "general medical-surgical experience" before deciding in what type of specialty nursing to ultimately settle, the implication being that M-S units were only a starting point to practice procedures, perform treatments, and build on skills taught in school, but not necessarily someplace a nurse would want to remain. Medical-surgical units have traditionally been regarded as the stepping stone to specialty areas such as pediatrics, oncology, cardiac, and renal units. Referring to these units as "special" care consciously or subconsciously implied to M-S nurses and the public that more important, out of the ordinary, or noteworthy care could be expected, as compared to basic, not special, or not noteworthy care provided in M-S units. Nurses who have chosen M-S as their area of practice have always found this rather perplexing and frustrating.

Concentrating patient populations based on age groups or diagnostic types simply means that care is directed toward, or limited to, particular and distinct age groups or diagnostic types. Nurses working on general M-S units traditionally cannot limit their knowledge and skills to any one particular patient type; rather, they are called on to amass broad knowledge, adeptness, and competence for numerous patient populations and a multiplicity of diagnoses. The purpose here is not to negate the various specializations within nursing, but rather to call for the recognition of M-S nursing as an area of specialization. And as an area of specialization, it has its own unique challenges and contributions to make, both for patient outcomes and for nursing practice.

The M-S environment has changed rapidly over time. Such influences as growing consumer involvement, alternate methods of care delivery, dwindling health dollars, increases in acuity, growth of minority populations and the poor, and advances in health care technology have highlighted and contributed to the diversity and complexity of M-S nursing. As a result, the M-S arena is finally being recognized and accepted as a unique and evolving specialty area.

As a specialty area, it has its unique contributions, challenges, and dilemmas for patient care and nursing practice. Nowhere is this better demonstrated than within QA activities.

QUALITY ASSURANCE IN TRANSITION

While quality assurance has undergone numerous transformations during the last century (Bull, 1985), it is sometimes difficult to see that any growth or progress has occurred. Discussions and debates still abound in practice and in the QA literature on exactly what product the health care industries are trying to produce, who the consumers of the product are, whose perspectives on quality should be considered, and whether the focus of quality assurance should be on the product, the individuals who produce the product, or the environment in which the product is produced. The various evaluation strategies and empirical studies that have emerged over time represent attempts to answer some of these questions (Lang & Clinton, 1984). No consensus on the "right way to do quality assurance" currently exists, or may even be possible or desirable, given the large number of variables and ambiguities involved in health care and nursing practice. However, through the combined efforts of consumers, payers, governmental agencies, health care providers, researchers, and accreditation agencies, such as the Joint Commission on Accreditation of Healthcare Organizations, more commonly accepted and agreed-on guidelines will evolve to assist those involved in the pursuit of quality health care and patient outcomes.

THE MONITORING AND EVALUATION PROCESS

Quality assurance in M-S units can be especially demanding due to the complexity and diversity of its population mix. Adherence to the Joint Commission requirements for monitoring and evaluating nursing care and patient outcomes at times seems unachievable, given this population. However, in exploring various ways in which M-S nurses have attempted to comply with the guidelines of the Joint Commission, a ten-step process for monitoring and evaluation may help identify common concerns and dilemmas and stimulate innovative and creative ideas for QA activities. Equally important is the realization that there is no one right way to meet Joint Commission standards; a variety of approaches is acceptable and encouraged (Patterson, personal communication, October 19, 1989).

Assign Responsibility

The overall responsibility for the QA program may be broadly stated in the hospital or nursing department/service QA plan. However, difficulties will arise for M-S units if this plan does not specifically assign or designate individuals responsible for each step of the QA process. The roles of staff nurses, unit-based QA members, unit managers, administrators, and other individuals involved in medical-surgical QA activities (i.e., staff development personnel, case managers, clinical nurse specialists, educators, etc.) must be clearly delineated.

Clear assignment of activities helps diminish the confusion, role uncertainty, and apathy that can result when accountability, responsibility, and authority are not specified. For example, who decides what clinical issues should be monitored on an M-S unit? Should it be staff nurses, unit managers, the QA coordinator, or the nursing department/service?

The intent of assigning responsibility should be approached from the perspective of which individual/group has the unique knowledge and skill needed to most effectively contribute or perform each step of the QA process. We all have a unique contribution to make to improving nursing care and patient outcomes.

Assigning responsibilities clearly articulates these domains. Exhibit 3-1 is an example of a nursing department QA plan and assignment of responsibilities.

Delineating the Scope of Service/Care

This step is intended to provide a complete inventory of what the unit does and may include conditions or diseases treated, therapies provided, procedures used, patient populations served, and professional disciplines providing services. Once delineated, the scope of service provides a basis for the subsequent steps of the monitoring and evaluation process.

While, in theory, this step should be relatively easy to complete, M-S nurses have expressed some difficulties and frustrations unique to this practice area. First, few examples are available in the literature to serve as references for M-S areas. On the one hand, examples currently available from the Joint Commission in its series on *Examples of Monitoring and Evaluating* (Joint Commission, 1988a, 1988b, 1988c) relate to specific areas of practice such as obstetrics and gynecology, emergency services, and "special" care (intensive care) units. Medical-surgical nurses may find that these Joint Commission examples are too specific to particular patient types (i.e., Caesarean sections, premature neonates, trauma patients, ventilation-supported patients) to be applicable to the divergent diagnostic mix and the varying activity levels and age groups seen on most M-S units. Clinical nursing QA literature, on the other hand, typically addresses specific elements of the QA process, such as program design (Clough & Hall, 1987; Marker, 1987; Nadzam & Atkins, 1987; Watson, Bulechek, & McCloskey, 1987; Westfall, 1987) or program evaluation (Deurr & Staats, 1988; Milton, 1988; Poster & Pelletier, 1988; Saum, 1988; Smeltzer, 1988). These examples do not usually incorporate the specific requirements of accrediting agencies such as the Joint Commission. Thus, nurses may feel there is never a meeting of the minds between Joint Commission and nursing literature.

Medical-surgical nurses have also expressed uncertainties regarding how inclusive or comprehensive to be in writing their scope of service. Should it be written solely by nurses and only from their perspective? Should other disciplines be involved? How much of the organizational design of the facility, if any, should be included? Should operating guidelines of the medical staff or bylaws be incorporated? Examples from the Joint Commission are ideally devised from an organizationwide approach for the care of patients in a particular environment (i.e., obstetrics, emergency, emergent, or critical care) and incorporate the contributions of multiple disciplines under the direction of a medical director. However, in typical M-S units, an organizationwide approach is difficult to take because nurses are usually the only ones attempting to write scopes of service for their areas. Various medical services are represented, and, thus, no *one* medical

Exhibit 3-1 A Nursing Department's QA Plan and Assignment of Responsibility

Scope: Nursing QA activities are integrated in all departments within the facility. Efforts are made to avoid duplication of activities and to utilize resources effectively. The plan is consistent with the goals and philosophy of the facility.

Purpose: To provide a comprehensive, ongoing, and systematic program to monitor and evaluate the quality and appropriateness of care, pursue opportunities to improve care, and resolve identified problems.

Objectives:

1. To identify important aspects of patient care activities and/or nursing practice that have the greatest importance/significance to the quality and appropriateness of patient care.
2. To develop indicators of care that reflect agreed-on acceptable levels of patient care or nursing practice for the important aspects of care.
3. To collect, review, and/or evaluate information on the quality and/or appropriateness of important aspects of care on an ongoing basis.
4. To initiate actions to resolve known or potential problems and/or to identify opportunities to improve care.
5. To document and report findings and conclusions of monitoring, evaluation, and problem-solving activities.
6. To participate in the integration of the hospital's QA program.

Organization:

1. The QA program is decentralized (unit-based); therefore, each unit manager is responsible for completing the activities necessary to achieve the objectives.
2. Each unit has a QA committee, comprised of staff nurses, the unit manager, and the clinical nurse specialist (CNS), that is responsible for completing the QA activities for the unit.
3. The QA Coordinating Committee, comprised of unit management, nursing administrators, staff nurses, clinical nurse specialists, and nurse educators, reviews and evaluates the overall QA activities for the department of nursing. Final recommendations are made to the director of nursing.
4. Results of QA activities are submitted to the facilitywide QA committee and the governing board.

QA Activity	*Responsible Person/Unit for Clinical Issues*	*Responsible Person/Dept. for Management Issues*
Identify important aspects of care	Unit QA staff nurses in consultation with CNS unit manager	Nurse managers with approval of director of nursing
Establish indicators of care and thresholds for action	Unit QA staff nurses in consultation with CNS and QA coordinator and unit manager	Nurse managers with approval of director of nursing
Collect and organize data	Unit QA committee members in conjunction with unit staff and medical records department	Departmental QA data to be collected by QA Coordinator and/or medical records department

Exhibit 3-1 continued

QA Activity	Responsible Person/Unit for Clinical Issues	Responsible Person/Dept. for Management Issues
Evaluate care when thresholds are met	Unit QA committee in conjunction with staff and unit management	Nursing Executive Committee in conjunction with unit managers
Take action	Unit QA committee in conjunction with staff and unit management	Director of nursing
Assess effectiveness of actions	Unit QA committee in conjunction with staff and unit management	Nursing Administration Committee in conjunction with unit managers
Communicate results	Unit QA committee in conjunction with unit manager	Report prepared by nursing QA Coordinator

director is accountable for all services provided by all disciplines. Medical-surgical nurses are not responsible for listing the activities of other disciplines, such as physicians, respiratory therapists, and social workers, in their scope of services since they are not accountable for them.

Scopes of care for M-S areas can range from short narratives to all-inclusive documents. Generally, however, M-S nurses prefer a short narrative that adequately relates an overall picture of what their area is like. This may include bed size, nurse staffing ratios and staff mix, age of patients, and modality of care delivery. Other factors include diagnostic types, treatments, procedures or care provided by nurses, and use of the nursing process. Delineating the scope of service is an ongoing process that needs to be modified as patient populations, services, care practices, or staffing ratios/mix are changed, added, or deleted. See Exhibit 3-2 for an example of the scope of service for a surgical unit, Exhibit 3-3 for an example of the authority and scope of service for a diabetic unit, and Exhibit 3-4 for an example of the scope of care/service for an M-S unit.

Important Aspects of Care

This step involves a more selective description of the M-S unit's (or nursing department's) therapeutic, supportive, palliative, preventive patient care activities that have the greatest impact on the quality and appropriateness of care and that are high risk, high volume, or problem prone (Patterson, 1988). Since it is neither practical nor useful to monitor all aspects of a particular unit's (or department's)

Exhibit 3-2 The Scope of Service for a Surgical Unit

---

4 West is a 28-bed acute care surgical unit that provides 24-hour nursing care to patients admitted for orthopedic, oral, or general surgical procedures. Orthopedic surgical intervention may include any bone fracture, joint replacement, and/or removal of a failed prosthesis. Oral surgery may include partial or full mouth extractions with vestibuloplasty to complex mandibular reconstruction. Accident cases and patients with oral cancer are also among the patients undergoing oral surgery. The most common general surgical procedure performed is inguinal hernia repair, but common procedures also include fistulae repair, post cava bypass, and gastric and colon resections.

The emphases for all surgical patients are preoperative instruction and close postoperative monitoring, which include

- wound and circulation management
- prevention of atelectasis
- accurate I & O
- monitoring of vital signs
- early ambulation
- pain control
- prevention of skin breakdown

Assessments upon admission are done to assure early discharge planning and community referrals for home care. Modified team nursing is utilized. The nursing staff consists of 10 RNs, 5 licensed practical nurses, and 3 nursing assistants. The head nurse is assisted by designated charge RNs for each shift.

Source: Adapted with permission of Veterans Administration Medical Center, Omaha, NE.

---

services, the current intent of this step is to focus monitoring and evaluation efforts on those activities that offer the greatest opportunity to improve patient care or nursing practice (Patterson, personal communication, October 19, 1989).

Many important aspects of care are possible focuses, depending on whose perspective is being considered: the clinical staff, the managers, or the nurse administrators. For example, clinicians on an M-S unit will be concerned with identifying *clinical* activities that relate to the hands-on or face-to-face interactions between the patient and the nurse, such as pain management, safe administration of medications, and timely and appropriate assessments and interventions. The nurse manager is concerned, over and above the clinical aspects, with *managerial* important aspects of care, such as adequate and appropriate staffing, sufficient supplies and equipment, and physical safety of the environment, and ongoing develoment of the staff. The nurse administrator has to ensure that adequate systems are in place to support clinical and management staff and to ascertain all

Exhibit 3-3 The Authority and Scope of Care for a Diabetic Unit

---

I. Authority:

The Nursing Manager/Supervisor of the Diabetic Unit will be responsible for the monitoring and evaluation activities. He/she will identify and define the responsibilities of the Diabetic Unit's Quality Assurance Committee. The committee is comprised of a chairman and the charge nurses on the 7–3 and 3–11 shifts. This committee, with staff input, is responsible for defining the Major Clinical Functions, Important Aspects of Care, and Indicators which comprise the monitoring program. They also are responsible for data collection, analysis, and evaluation with the assistance of the entire professional staff. They have the responsibility for and authority to take action to resolve identified problems with input and approval of the Manager/Supervisor.

II. Scope of Care:

This unit is a 20-bed medical-surgical area with an emphasis on the diabetic patient. The staff is comprised of RNs, licensed practical nurses, nursing assistants, and a nurse diabetes educator.

Initial and ongoing assessments of patients' knowledge/skills are conducted regarding what diabetes is, diet, self-care habits, medication administration, hypo- or hyperglycemia, blood glucose monitoring, urine testing, and exercise. Physicians' and nurses' orders are carried out through the steps of the nursing process. An individualized diabetic care plan is utilized for directing patient care.

In coordination with the diabetes educators, staff provides patient/family education specific to diabetes and other coexisting diseases/illnesses. Discharge planning is coordinated with the Clinical Management department. Administration and monitoring of medications and IV therapy are a component of care. Assistance with activities of daily living is an aspect of care along with coordination of these activities with ancillary departments. Emotional support is provided to patients and families to assist in adaptation to their illness/disease process.

Major clinical functions identified through this scope of care include diabetes education, discharge planning, medication administration, infection control, nursing process, safety, maintenance of skin integrity, nutrition/fluid balance, pain management, and consumer satisfaction.

Source: Courtesy of Archbishop Bergan Mercy Hospital, Omaha, NE.

---

units are given fair and equitable treatment in the areas of resource allocation and utilization. Examples of *system* important aspects of care for the nurse administrator could include standards of care and performance, policies and procedures, development of the nursing staff, and research activities/utilization. Unit-specific aspects of care, as well as common aspects of care for the department, need to be considered.

One could argue that any one of the clinical, managerial, or system important aspects of care listed above could occur frequently, could put patients at high risk

Exhibit 3-4 The Authority and Scope of Care for a Medical-Surgical Unit

---

I. Authority:
   The Nursing Manager of 3 East will be responsible for monitoring and the evaluation activities. He/she will identify and define the responsibilities of the 3 East Quality Assurance Committee. The committee is comprised of a chairman and the charge nurses on the 7–3 and 3–11 shifts. This committee, with staff input, is responsible for defining the Major Clinical Functions, Important Aspects of Care, and Indicators which comprise the monitoring program. They are also responsible for data collection, analysis, and evaluation with the assistance of the entire professional staff. They have the responsibility for and authority to take action to resolve identified problems with input and approval of the Manager.

II. Scope of Care:
   3 East is a 31-bed medical-surgical unit with a staff comprised of RNs, licensed practical nurses, and nursing assistants. The major types of patients seen include cardiovascular, pulmonary, neurological, and urological.
   Initial and ongoing assessments of patients are conducted. Physicians' and nurses' orders are carried out through the steps of the nursing process. Policies, procedures, standards, infection control, and safety practices are used as guidelines for care delivery. Staff provides patient/family education specific to the disease process/treatment. Discharge planning is coordinated with the Clinical Management department. Administration and monitoring of medications and IV therapy are a chief component of care. Assistance with activities of daily living is provided along with coordination of these activities with ancillary departments. Emotional support is provided to patients and families to assist in adaptation to their illness/disease process.
   The major clinical functions identified through this scope of care include the nursing process, safety, infection control, patient/family education, discharge planning, medication administration, pain management, nutrition/fluid balance, maintenance of skin integrity, and consumer satisfaction.

Source: Courtesy of Archbishop Bergan Mercy Hospital, Omaha, NE.

---

if not provided, or could be prone to cause problems for patients or staff. All of these clinical, managerial, and administrative examples are components of any comprehensive QA program that includes process, outcome, and structure orientations. However, the focus of *clinical* important aspects of care should be on the *clinical* elements perceived by M-S nurses to be most critical for patients to receive, not on the managerial or administrative aspects. Nursing is a practice discipline, and, therefore, M-S staff nurses, as experts in the clinical area, should have the strongest voice in determining the important aspects of care for their respective areas. In a centralized QA program, staff representatives from various clinical areas should be involved in determining common aspects of care for the department, as well as any specific aspects of care unique to their practice area.

The difficulty experienced by M-S nurses in identifying important aspects of care flowing from comprehensive scopes of care is that an inexhaustible laundry list usually results. To nurses, all things are important for certain patients at one point or another! Nurses educated to be holistic in dealing with the total patient face dilemmas when asked to identify and then prioritize "pieces" of the patient. Many M-S nurses shun the traditional medical model that focuses on important aspects of care related to diagnostic categories or disease entities, such as management of the patient with congestive heart failure, care of the insulin-dependent diabetic, or management of the oncology patient. Nurses may wonder if there are some common denominators that would cross all diagnostic lines. Among those common denominators identified in the literature and in practice are pain management, safety, patient education, discharge preparation, psychosocial support, and provision of basic human needs such as nutrition, hydration, elimination, and cleanliness.

Considering important aspects of care that focus on treatments or procedures performed, such as medication administration, suctioning, intravenous care, telemetry monitoring, administration of blood products, and dressing changes, can be equally disturbing to M-S nurses. The emphasis here is on "things" necessary to monitor or support the physical requirements of care. These things may represent another fragmentation of the patient into divisible parts, and many M-S nurses find this foreign to their value system.

Identifying problem-prone areas for important aspects of care can pose difficulties for M-S nurses. Items such as readmission to the M-S unit, nosocomial infection rates, stat lab or medication orders, education of the elderly patient for home management, and documentation in the medical record all could be considered problem-prone areas for most M-S environments. However, M-S nurses may hesitate to honestly identify them as such because they believe they will not be able to solve or improve care based solely on nursing interventions. Variables such as patient compliance, severity of illness, lack of communication between disciplines, and system problems are not directly controllable by M-S nurses. If they cannot fix them or improve them, nurses may avoid identifying them in the first place. Ignoring issues because they are difficult problems to solve is not acceptable. Efforts should be made with the resources that are available to identify and to solve or improve issues that have the greatest impact for patient outcomes or practice. This may be accomplished by working on smaller pieces of the problem, rather than by trying to solve the entire problem at one time.

To identify important aspects of care having the greatest impact on patient outcomes is a definite challenge to all nurses. Traditionally, we have looked at tangible elements of care that are easier to identify, quantify, and measure, such as physical assessments, patient education, or medication errors. While these elements are certainly important, they do not adequately present the whole picture of quality patient care. Something seems to be missing.

The missing piece may be the patients themselves. What do patients believe about quality care? Hays (1987) reported on a national survey of 4,000 consumers in which 52 percent mentioned employees' caring attitudes as an attribute associated with high-quality care. Steiber (1988) reported on a national poll in which 414 consumers denoted that satisfaction with the hospital experience was influenced more by concern shown than by clinical care.

The elements of caring and concern are not foreign to nurses. In fact, caring and concern are universally accepted and valued as being the "art" of professional nursing practice. These elements relay to patients the feeling of dignity and respect for their personal sense of well-being.

If patients do associate caring and concern as being most important to their perceptions of quality care, then nurses would be wise to identify care and concern as important aspects of care within their quality assurance programs. This may seem to be a difficult if not impossible task because caring and concern are viewed as intangible and nonquantifiable terms. However, continued efforts must be made to better examine, define, and articulate the meaning of caring and concern to patient satisfaction and their importance on positive patient outcomes.

In practice, M-S nurses often write a broad, but comprehensive, initial list of all things considered to be important for care. The list is then narrowed, and commonly agreed-on values are prioritized. These prioritized values usually appear in their final written document. Without this narrowing and prioritizing, M-S nurses tend to feel all elements identified need to be monitored and evaluated, creating an unrealistic and unachievable QA nightmare. Starting small with only one or two important aspects of care seems to help M-S nurses understand the intent of the Joint Commission requirement and fosters realistic expectations for continuing improvement of care. See Exhibit 3-5 for an example of a diabetic unit's important aspects of care and Exhibit 3-6 for an example of an M-S unit's important aspects of care.

Exhibit 3-5 The Important Aspects of Care for a Diabetic Unit

1. Nursing management of the newly diagnosed diabetic (high risk, problem prone)
2. Management of the nutritional needs of the diabetic patient (high volume, problem prone)
3. Pre- and postmanagement of the diabetic patient undergoing surgery/procedure (high volume, problem prone)
4. Management of the patient with hypoglycemia (high risk)
5. Management of the diabetic patient undergoing eye surgery (high risk, problem prone)

Source: Courtesy of Archbishop Bergan Mercy Hospital, Omaha, NE.

Exhibit 3-6 The Important Aspects of Care for a Medical-Surgical Unit

---

1. Management of the patient post-TURP (high volume)
2. Nursing management of the patient with dementia (high risk, high volume, problem prone)
3. Nursing management of the patient with a CVA (high risk, high volume, problem prone)
4. Care of the patient with MS (high volume, problem prone)
5. Care of the patient with respiratory-related illnesses (high risk, high volume, problem prone)
6. Consumer satisfaction

Source: Courtesy of Archbishop Bergan Mercy Hospital, Omaha, NE.

Indicators of Care

The QA chapter in the *1990 Accreditation Manual for Hospitals* specifies indicators to be developed for the important aspects of care and may include clinical criteria (standards of care, standards of practice, guidelines, or parameters). These indicators need to be objective, measurable, and based on current knowledge and to reflect structure, processes, and outcomes of care (Joint Commission, 1989b). An indicator can also include all three elements of structure, process, and outcome to measure one important aspect of care (Patterson, 1988).

This step of the Joint Commission's ten-step process seems to cause more confusion and frustration for M-S nurses than any other step. Several reasons exist for this. First, the term *indicator* is new and has not been part of the nursing QA model developed by Dr. Norma Lang, adopted by the American Nurses' Association, and utilized in practice since the 1970s (Bull, 1985; Lieske, 1985). Second, few examples of indicators are currently available in the literature to serve as reference points or guidelines for M-S nurses who are trying to develop their own unit-specific indicators. Some may prefer to maintain the status quo and "wait for Joint Commission to tell us what they want." Third, the Joint Commission's published examples of possible indicators are viewed by many nurses as based on the medical model and centered primarily on documentation, morbidity-mortality, and complications. Fourth, nursing and hospital QA coordinators, managers, and administrators may not understand the direction and intent of the Joint Commission Agenda for Change, the evolutionary process that needs to occur, or the steps necessary to meet the Joint Commission QA standards. Thus, the leaders themselves may not be knowledgeable enough to assist the staff in developing indicators of care. Mixed, confusing, or uninformed directions given by these individuals can result in a conflict of values, lost time, and a feeling by M-S staff nurses that nobody knows what they are doing.

Fifth, confusion in definitions and usage of such terms as *standards, indicators, criteria, parameters for care, protocols,* and *studies* exists in the practice areas and in the literature. This nonagreement of terms can cause disharmony because nurses are not able to speak the same language. What some nurses call standards, others call important aspects of care; some refer to indicators as standards; and some nurses call indicators (or subindicators) criteria. For example, is "the patient can verbalize knowledge of discharge medications by dismissal" a standard or an indicator? Should the same example be written in more measurable terms: ". . . to include (1) medication name (2) dosage, and (3) side effects"? Are these qualifiers then called criteria or indicators/subindicators? The answer to the above question depends on the written definitions of terms that need to be in place for each facility, as well as the guidelines for how these terms are to be utilized. The Joint Commission encourages a wide variety of options in developing indicators. As long as an M-S unit identifies measurable statements that are believed to reflect the most high-volume, high-risk, or problem-prone issues on that unit, the intent of the Joint Commission requirement for indicators will be met. The exact mechanism is left up to us.

Last, well-defined indicators are difficult to develop because of the very nature of most M-S units. The wide variety of patient types and subspecialties does not lend itself very easily to a prioritization of what is most important to monitor and evaluate. As a result, nurses may develop rather lengthy lists when developing indicators, such as the following:

Important Aspect of Care: Patient teaching in preparation for discharge

Indicators:
1. Assessments include
   a. current knowledge level
   b. ability to understand instructions
   c. physical and mental handicaps
   d. acceptance level for present illness
   e. living conditions
   f. financial status
   g. coping mechanism utilized
   h. availability of support services
2. The patient/family can describe planned home care including
   a. treatment/procedures
   b. prescribed medication (name, purpose, dose, schedule)
   c. diet restrictions
   d. physical care
   e. activity level
3. Necessary supplies for immediate home care are provided.

4. The patient is informed of available community resources necessary for home care.

This example really contains four indicators. The first and second indicators contain eight and five subindicators (or criteria, depending on the definitions used), respectively. Nothing is inherently wrong with this list *if* ample staffing, time, and resources are in place for timely data collection. However, the majority of M-S units are not so blessed, and consideration should be given to reducing the number of indicators to those viewed as most important, such as the following:

1. Patient knowledge of self-care needs is assessed throughout hospitalization.
2. The patient can verbalize medication name, dose, and schedule by dismissal.
3. Community referrals are made according to established guidelines and patient needs.

Or perhaps the above three indicators would need further simplification because of the time needed to extract the data from the medical record. The resulting indicators could be the following:

1. Potential patient needs for discharge are documented on admission.
2. The discharge instruction sheet is signed by the patient on dismissal.

Medical-surgical nurses would benefit from starting with only one or two indicators that are manageable in terms of nurses' time, resources, and staffing. Starting small has other benefits as well. For example, data collection for these two indicators could easily be conducted by staff nurses. Attention to only two specific areas, admission assessments and the discharge sheet, focuses the effort and allows for realistic opportunities for improvement to occur. Limiting indicators also lessens the anxiety and frustration that commonly result with a laundry list of multiple indicators.

In summary, the area of indicator development for M-S nurses is a new and evolving phenomenon. Many unknowns exist and have caused confusion and apprehension in the practice area. Numerous concerns and possible barriers to effective indicator development need to be identified and addressed by M-S nurses in order to reduce their levels of anxiety and frustration.

Quality assurance coordinators, nurse managers, and administrators need to become better informed about the requirements of the Joint Commission QA standards as well as the possible barriers to successful implementation of the standards in clinical practice. With this knowledge, they are better prepared to guide M-S nurses and help them realize their creative and innovative potential for appropriate indicator development.

Establish Thresholds for Evaluation

Most M-S nurses feel relief at having the flexibility to establish realistic thresholds that are not all set at 100 percent or 0 percent. These ideal percentages, while always the goal, are something only rarely achieved. For example, saying that all newly diagnosed diabetics will be knowledgeable and able to care for themselves by dismissal 100 percent of the time is unrealistic. Patients are simply not emotionally or mentally able to absorb during short hospital stays all that they must know to adequately care for themselves. Realistically, teaching and care can begin only while the patient is hospitalized, and they need to be supplemented and reinforced beyond dismissal. Thus, revising this indicator may be necessary.

Any data from unit-specific trends could be used in establishing thresholds. Hospital-specific, regional, or national norms, when available, could also be utilized (American Hospital Association, 1989). Examples include readmission rates, nosocomial infection rates, fall rates, medication error rates, and percentages of patients receiving certain treatments or procedures such as tube feedings, parenteral therapy, and chemotherapy. In the absence of comparative data, the M-S staff nurses should use their clinical experience and better judgment to set the initial threshold and then adjust that threshold as comparative data become available.

For example, M-S nurses may desire to maintain skin integrity for orthopedic patients and, thus, set the threshold at 95 percent. At first glance, the threshold may seem appropriate. However, if the general patient population base consists of individuals whose skin integrity was already compromised on admission, such as those with diabetes, alcoholism, liver dysfunction, or nutritional deficits, or if patients are admitted with decubitus ulcers already present, then the threshold of 95 percent may be unrealistic. If unit-specific data were available, the nurses could be given some assistance in setting thresholds. As a hypothetical example, if a nurse collected data over time and determined 25 percent of the orthopedic patients had altered skin integrity on admission, another 1–2 percent experienced worsening of the skin integrity during hospitalization, and the average length of stay was five days, the threshold might be more realistically set at 80–85 percent. Improving skin integrity for 26–27 percent of the normal population base within five days simply may not be possible. The judgment of M-S staff is essential in determining thresholds that directly relate to clinical issues. Managerial staff can assist by gathering or presenting background data and information on the particular indicator under discussion.

In some instances, M-S nurses may want to have a threshold of 0 percent or 100 percent, especially if the indicator describes a serious complication or outcome. Setting a threshold at 0 percent or 100 percent means that even one deviation will merit a thorough investigation. Examples include mismanagement of chemotherapy agents, mechanical restraints inappropriately applied, and inadequate monitoring or reporting of unstable vital signs.

In practice, M-S nurses may have a tendency to initially set thresholds too high and be reluctant to redirect them to more realistic levels, even when legitimate comparative data become available and in-depth investigations do not reveal a problem or an opportunity to improve care. Somehow, lowering the threshold may be perceived as lowering the standards of care for patients or as denying that nurses should be able to do all things for all patients. Making legitimate adjustments in thresholds is appropriate and necessary and avoids poor utilization of scarce resources.

Another question often raised by M-S nurses is whether each individual indicator should have its own threshold or whether one threshold is adequate for several indicators. For example:

Important Aspect of Care: Preoperative teaching of patients undergoing radical mastectomy

Indicators:

1. Patients can demonstrate turning, coughing, and deep-breathing techniques prior to surgery.
2. Patient knowledge of planned surgical intervention is documented.
3. Family members are aware of the location of the surgery waiting room.

The decision to set one overall threshold or individual thresholds for each indicator should be based on several considerations, including the unit-specific or patient population variables normally seen (i.e., age, anxiety level, family support, knowledge level, admission date in relation to surgery date, resources, etc.). However, the greatest consideration needs to be given to the risk involved if the particular indicator is not fulfilled. Perhaps all indicators do not carry an equal risk. In the above example, the first and second indicators may be judged to be more crucial for the patients' postoperative course; thus, setting individual thresholds at (1) 89 percent, (2) 90 percent, and (3) 75 percent, respectively, is appropriate.

Indicators believed to carry equal risk or to be valued equally could denote one threshold for all indicators.

Important Aspect of Care: Management of patients receiving blood products (packed cells or whole blood)

Indicators (*THRESHOLD*—100 percent):

1. Packed cells are checked by two RNs prior to administration.
2. Vital signs are checked immediately prior to administration and every 5 minutes for the first 15 minutes of administration.
3. The patient is assessed every 15 minutes for signs of a possible transfusion reaction.
4. The transfusion is stopped and the physician notified immediately if a transfusion reaction is suspected.

Setting thresholds does require reflective thought. In the absence of comparative data or trends, valuable clinical experience and professional judgment can help M-S nurses set thresholds that are realistic and achievable. [See Exhibits 3-7 through 3-9 for examples of thresholds established for indicators (subindicators/criteria) for important aspects of care.] Most thresholds are set relatively high, however, because of the need to devote scarce nursing time to high-priority indicators.

Collect and Organize Data

The standards listed in the *1990 Accreditation Manual for Hospitals* (Joint Commission, 1989b) require data to be collected for each indicator. How many to include (sample size) and how often to collect (data collection frequency) are dependent on three relevant and rational principles: how often the event/activity occurs, how important or significant the event/activity is, and how long the event/activity has been problemfree (Joint Commission, 1989).

This flexibility in sampling size and data collection frequency allows M-S nurses to realistically plan and utilize their resources efficiently. The Joint Commission does not mandate a specific number for sample size, but provides a general guideline of 20 cases or 5 percent, whichever is greater (Patterson, 1989). The purpose of sampling, according to Polit and Hungler (1987), is to select a portion of the population to represent the entire population.

Sampling every activity/event is generally not indicated or realistic in QA. It is more economical and practical to work with smaller numbers, and it is usually possible to obtain an understanding of the event being investigated (Polit & Hungler, 1987). The main consideration in identifying and studying a sample is how well it represents or approximates the population from which it was chosen. One is concerned with patterns or trends, not individual cases. A few instances do exist that would necessitate that data be collected on all activities/events in a given population. These may include indicators that occur very infrequently, but are a high risk to patients, or any indicators that have thresholds set at 0 percent or 100 percent. In these instances, one is concerned about individual cases, not patterns or trends.

Medical-surgical nurses may have difficulty determining adequate sample sizes, even with the general guideline of 5 percent or 20 cases, because they may not consider the frequency of the data collection and data evaluation intervals. For example, are 5 percent or 20 cases to be sampled per week, per month, or per quarter? How is this to be determined? Will the data be evaluated monthly or quarterly? All of these elements need to be considered in order to not overburden staff nurses and to make the best use of limited resources. A variety of options is available. If, for example, nurses on a 40-bed orthopedic unit decide to monitor patient ability to crutch walk on dismissal, what would be a realistic sample size, monitoring frequency, and evaluation frequency? It is determined 75 percent of this population (or 30 patients) are generally dismissed with crutches and a patient's usual length of stay is one week. Thus, 30 patients per week times 4 weeks would yield 120 possible patients to monitor per month. Five percent of 120 is six patients—which may not be an adequate number to evaluate; thus, data on 20 cases a month would initially be collected in order to do a monthly evaluation.

Is it always necessary to collect data on 20 patients a month or to evaluate this data monthly? Probably not. Routinely collecting data on 6 or 7 random patients a month and evaluating the composite data on a quarterly basis may be more realistic and manageable. This assumption is based on the high volume of patients dismissed with crutches and consideration for the significance of crutch walking for patient outcomes. Establishing hard and fast rules on the sample size, data collection frequency, and evaluation frequency would not be practical or desirable in most cases. Multiple inherent variables would need to be explained for each indicator. The above illustration of monitoring patients' ability to crutch walk by dismissal would need to be reconsidered in different situations or environments. For example, units with smaller numbers would need to adjust their sample size or their monitoring frequency. Units experiencing readmissions of patients over 65 years of age due to falls resulting from an inability to crutch walk on dismissal may need to monitor and evaluate all such cases. Units showing no problems or opportunities to improve care could decrease the frequency of monitoring and evaluation—or discontinue them all together.

Sometimes M-S nurses collect and evaluate data according to set schedules established by the nursing department, hospital QA committee, or other organizational authorities. Weekly monitoring and monthly evaluation, monthly data reviews and evaluation, and monthly data collection and quarterly evaluation are the mandated frequencies usually seen. While establishing such schedules may be indicated and necessary in some situations, they may not be practical or relevant for all situations. They may be rules applied without consideration of the frequency or the significance of the event/activity monitored. Set rules also may not consider the time or resources needed to implement the effective system changes necessary to solve problems or to improve care. For example, if ongoing monitoring reveals a problem correctable by establishing new policies, hiring a consultant, or modifying orientation or inservice procedures, these changes need to occur before monitoring is resumed. To require continued monitoring before the corrective action or intervention has occurred is not only a waste of time and resources, but also extremely frustrating for staff nurses.

Another dilemma evident with mandated data collection and evaluation frequencies is that adequate and reliable information may not be obtainable in the time allocated. Required ongoing monthly reviews and evaluations of all patients with mechanical restraints (in the absence of an identified problem) may yield a very low sample on which an evaluation can be based. More reliable data would be needed for M-S nurses to intelligently identify trends or to evaluate the quality and appropriateness of care.

Sometimes, in the rush to demonstrate ongoing monitoring, data collection methodologies may not be appropriately selected. For example, a monthly retrospective review of ten medical records, with a quarterly compilation of data to evaluate the adequacy of discharge diabetic teaching, would require a fair amount of time each month to complete. Would not the same information be obtained through quarterly review of 20 random medical records (or 5 percent of diabetic patients) representing all three months of the quarter? Data collection would still be ongoing, but in a manner that would utilize staff time more efficiently for evaluation of the data.

Once data are collected, they should be organized in such a way that trends in care or opportunities for improvement are readily identifiable. This can be accomplished in a variety of ways. Graphic displays such as histograms, bar graphs, statistical tables, and line graphs can be used to supplement and clarify a narrative report (Lieske, 1985). Data can also be presented by the use of a form that compares the desired performance (thresholds) to the actual performance (thresholds). Narrative summaries alone are acceptable, but can become lengthy and pose difficulties in presenting the data in a factual and an objective manner. Regardless of the format selected, the data need to be clear, explicit, and complete so that M-S nurses can determine if further evaluation is indicated.

Evaluate Care When Thresholds Are Reached

An evaluation of the quality and appropriateness of care is necessary when results of the data are at variance with the established threshold for action (Joint Commission, 1989b). This evaluation is intended to be an in-depth review to examine trends, identify specifics when the cause and scope of a problem are unknown, or to ascertain further information that may help identify ways to improve care. Unexplained or unacceptable variances in care necessitate that energy be focused on evaluating why the variances occurred. The evaluation includes even single important events (Joint Commission, 1989b).

Medical-surgical staff nurses are experts in utilizing assessment and evaluation skills on their own individual patients. They are aware that multiple reasons may exist for a patient's problems and have numerous options to offer the patient on how these problems may be reduced or resolved. The same analysis and creativity used by nurses to evaluate patient care need to be transferred into the arena of quality assurance.

In practice, M-S staff nurses may perform this step of analysis too quickly, without carefully interpreting the data. Nurses can be swift to blame themselves for all the variances found and fail to realize other real possibilities exist.

Varying degrees of rigor exist in evaluating/analyzing the data—from simple to complex. How much rigor to apply will depend on how much information is needed to interpret the data accurately and objectively. For example, if the data reveal preoperative patients are not receiving preoperative teaching information, the reason can be very simple. The supply of booklets could have been depleted due to budget cutbacks. Or an evaluation of the medical record of a patient who sustained a fractured hip as a result of a fall may show that all possible precautions were appropriately taken. Nothing humanly possible could have been done to prevent the fall. In such cases, continued monitoring is the only thing that can realistically be done. Evaluation can also be complex, as when determining the reason for an increase in medication errors. Questions such as these need to be asked: Is there really an increase, or are trends reflective of the fact that more medications are being given than in the past? Who is making the errors? What types of errors are being made? Why? Multiple reasons may exist for which data have not been collected. Further data would be needed before knowledgeable evaluation can occur.

Medical-surgical staff nurses should determine if the data presented are valid and reliable. Do they reflect what they were supposed to measure? Is the sample size adequate to reflect trends? Can the results be trusted to be true? Was the data collection methdology appropriate? If the answer to any of these questions is no, further energy should be directed to rectifying these concerns before steps are taken to resolve problems identified on the basis of potentially inaccurate data. If, for example, data from four patients' medical records reveal that knowledge of discharge medication is poor, one should question the small sample size, whether patient knowledge was really deficient, and whether the documentation of such was really the concern.

After the data have been judged to be valid and reliable, M-S nurses should try to determine if any patterns or trends are evident. Is the concern related to a particular nurse or group of nurses? Is it occurring on all shifts or at particular times? Does it involve selected pieces of equipment or documentation forms?

Does it apply to all patients or to a particular group of patients? Exploring these questions helps identify areas where further data collection may be needed to clarify the cause of the problem or opportunities to improve care.

The cause of the problem or area of concern must be clearly and appropriately identified before corrective actions can be taken. If problems are not clearly identified, the corrective action may have little or no effect on solving them.

In summary, when ongoing monitoring of care shows that a problem or opportunity to improve care exists, an in-depth evaluation needs to be conducted. This evaluation should include identifying whether the cause of the problem is attributable to a knowledge, performance, or system deficiency (Fournies, 1988; Magin & Pipe, 1990). Corrective actions can then logically flow from this framework.

Take Actions To Improve Care or Resolve Problems

Devising action plans can be difficult or impossible for M-S nurses if they have not adequately evaluated/analyzed the problem. When evaluation is carried out and the cause of the problem clearly identified, the necessary corrective action should become self-evident. If the action is not appropriate to the cause, little long-term change can be expected.

Nurses often develop action plans for what they perceive to be staff knowledge deficiencies when, in fact, only about 15 percent of all QA problems are attributable to lack of education or knowledge (Patterson, 1989). When knowledge or skill deficiencies are identified, a variety of appropriate ways exist to assist nurses in developing or reinforcing the needed skill. See Exhibit 3-7 for possible actions to solve or improve knowledge deficiencies.

Devising action plans for performance deficiencies can be more challenging because they most appropriately require intervention by the M-S nurse manager. Medical-surgical staff nurses should avoid trying to implement any corrective action involving individual nurses. Such corrective action is appropriate, however, when broad performance problems relate to the unit or groups of nurses. Performance can be positively affected by staff nurses through role modeling and providing feedback to peers regarding their skills or care of patients. See Exhibit 3-8 for possible actions to solve or improve performance deficiencies.

Formulating action plans for system, structure, or environmental deficiencies requires M-S nurses to seriously explore or re-examine what can be manipulated or changed within the system. Only then will they be able to provide care that is of better quality, is cost effective, and makes better use of time and personnel.

Action plan development can be facilitated by initially listing numerous options possible for resolving the problem or improving care—even far-fetched or "crazy" ideas. The goal is to solicit creative ideas that may not have been tried

Exhibit 3-7 Possible Actions to Solve or Improve Knowledge Deficiencies

• Attend workshop/seminar	• Offer 1:1 training/education
• Revise orientation information	• Arrange for "expert" guest speaker
• Provide mentors/facilitators	• Provide information from books or articles
• Provide an inservice	• Stress expectations or consequences
• Attend a course or class	• Provide opportunities to practice deficient skills
• Provide continuing education	• Develop self-learning packets
• Establish mutually set goals	• Use audiovisual material
• Develop policy, procedure, standards, or protocols	• Utilize skill inventories
• Confer with staff to determine the best method to develop knowledge/skill	

before or new ways of implementing old ideas. After the list is complete, begin group identification of those ideas having the greatest merit. Eventually, the group should arrive at an action plan necessary to improve care. Many ideas will be practical and realistic, such as consolidating flow sheets, revising policies and procedures, and developing printed material to assist in patient education. Others, hopefully, will be rather nontraditional and will cause nurses to seriously question their own habits, such as allowing competent patients to take their own medica-

Exhibit 3-8 Possible Actions to Solve or Improve Performance Deficiencies

• Encourage people to develop potential	• Remove any obstacles causing nonperformance
• Communicate expectations and goals for unit and individuals	• Arrange some time off for personal problems, if indicated
• Coach or counsel those who do not meet expectations	• Establish employee recognition programs
• Observe performance personally	• Role model expected performance
• Provide prompt positive/negative feedback	• Maintain open and honest communication with staff at all times
• Find ways (rewards) to strengthen desired behavior	• Post positive letters from patients on bulletin boards
• Communicate priorities	• Transfer or terminate
• Remove rewards for poor performance	• Develop detailed job descriptions
• Use negative consequences for nonperformance	• Suggest counseling by a professional for personal problems

tions (they will have to at home) or designating time frames (with management coverage of the unit) to allow and encourage timely care planning or documentation.

In summary, a variety of appropriate action plans can exist depending on the identified cause of the problem or concern. See Exhibit 3-9 for possible actions to solve or improve system deficiencies. Medical-surgical managers need to be instrumental, not defensive, in encouraging their staff to make suggestions for improvement. If nurses are afraid to offer suggestions or are put down when they do, they will not make them. Open and meaningful dialogue is necessary to overcome fear and to develop creative options to solve problems or improve care.

To effectively implement the change process, staff nurses must be involved. Assuring quality care implies that change may be needed in knowledge, performance or systems. Nurses need to be active participants in this change process (Kaye, 1988).

Assess Effectiveness of Action Plans and Document Improvement

Continued monitoring will indicate if the problem is resolving/resolved or if care is improved. Sometimes M-S nurses become overly anxious to see a "quick fix," once their action plans are implemented. However, changing care practices or outcomes of care may take time and patience. Altering learned behaviors, both in individuals and in systems, may take weeks or even months to logically occur. For example, when implementing a computerized care planning system based on nursing diagnoses, nurses will need time to become familiar with and effectively utilize the system. Just because immediate change did not occur does not mean the corrective action will not work.

If continued monitoring does not show improvement over time, M-S staff nurses should reassess whether the scope and cause of the problem were correctly

---

Exhibit 3-9 Possible Actions To Solve or Improve System Deficiencies

- Redesign delivery systems
- Create/revise forms
- Purchase/lease equipment
- Adjust inventories/supplies
- Formulate/revise policy or procedure
- Adjust staffing levels or ratios
- Seek services of a consultant/expert
- Revise job descriptions
- Redesign organizational structure
- Alter communication systems
- Eliminate unnecessary policies or other hindrances
- Computerize systems

identified, whether the actions taken to resolve the problem were appropriate and achievable, and whether the actions were implemented.

How long to monitor an indicator of care that is not a sentinel event (i.e., one that should always be monitored even with consistent high performance or outcomes) is not currently specified by the Joint Commission. Logically, it should be followed long enough to assure or validate that problem resolution or improved care resulted. Consideration should be given to the amount and type of data collected as well as the nature of the problem or concern and the particulars of the involved M-S unit. For example, monitoring the effectiveness of a falls prevention program may necessitate monthly monitoring until acceptable levels are achieved and then biyearly monitoring to assure levels are maintained. Or if a new flow sheet was devised that consolidated several forms, monitoring for three to six months should provide data sufficient to validate that the problem in recording physical parameters is resolved.

Communicate Results of Monitoring and Evaluation Activities

The final step of the Joint Commission process requires that findings, conclusions, recommendations, and actions taken and their effectiveness be recorded and reported to appropriate parties (Joint Commission, 1989b).

A variety of ways are utilized by M-S nurses to report QA findings; the final choice is dependent on the guidelines issued by either the nursing department or the organizational QA program. For example, the nursing department may require that M-S units maintain in-depth information, but that only overall narratives be presented on a quarterly basis. The organizationwide QA committee may require quarterly reporting of overall thresholds, with narratives addressing only those indicators that did not meet thresholds.

Generally, information is condensed as it proceeds up the administrative ladder. Medical-surgical nurses are not usually involved in this process in larger acute care facilities.

CONCLUSION

Major changes in the health care environment in recent years have transformed the general M-S units into areas of "specialization" for a wide variety of patient populations with a multiplicity of diagnoses or problems. Monitoring and evaluating nursing practice and patient care have also evolved through numerous stages of growth in determining the most effective way to perform QA activities, both in clinical practice and within the Joint Commission.

Numerous other changes can be expected as we move into the era of the 1990s. Nursing roles will continue to evolve through such innovations as case management/managed care, shared governance, and professional practice models. Our health care environment will become more data-driven as computer usage increases. The demand for professional nurses is expected to continue in comparison to the supply, requiring adjustments in the staff mix for many units. The necessity for multidisciplinary QA will become more evident as the acuity and complexity of patient care continue to rise. Such issues as costing out nursing services, addressing ethical concerns within nursing quality assurance, combining research and quality assurance, incorporating nursing diagnosis and nursing process into quality assurance and articulating important aspects of care will continue to be identified and explored.

What will be the challenges to M-S nurses in light of these numerous anticipated changes? How will these changes impact on the future evaluation of care? Nurses will need to thoughtfully consider what is really most important to patient outcomes and nursing practice. They can accomplish this through continued efforts to develop and clarify standards of care and standards of practice. One cannot rationally attempt to monitor and evaluate the quality of care that is not first defined. Research and QA interaction and dialogue will continue, thus increasing the value of tools used in quality assurance for data collection.

Medical-surgical nurses can increase efforts to motivate and sustain the commitment to quality assurance on their units, in essence assuring that nurses who provide patient care remain accountable and responsible for that care. Meaningful staff involvement will make quality assurance an integral part of care—not a separate entity. Creative ways to involve staff in light of diminishing resources are urgently needed. Staff nurse involvement is an essential component of quality assurance that cannot be negated.

Stronger support from M-S nurse managers can assist M-S nurses in taking nontraditional "risks" when devising and implementing actions to improve care or practice. Encouraging nurses to try new approaches can save valuable time, money, and energy. These efforts need to be fostered in order to achieve the greatest goals for quality.

Medical-surgical nurses, by the very nature of their practice environments, are flexible, innovative, and creative. Although the anticipated changes within quality assurance at times seem overwhelming, M-S nurses will no doubt respond to the challenges presented to them. When staff take the responsibility for quality assurance, the best overall improvements in patient outcomes and quality of care can be realized.

REFERENCES

American Hospital Association. (1989). *Technical briefing: The Joint Commission quality assurance model* (Technical Report). Chicago: Division of Quality Control Management, American Hospital Association.

Bull, M. (1985). Quality assurance: Its origins, transformations, and prospects. In C. Meisenheimer (Ed.), *Quality assurance—a complete guide to effective programs* (pp. 6–8). Rockville, MD: Aspen Publishers.

Clough, J., & Hall, K. (1987). Writing institutional criteria sets for nursing diagnosis: From idea to implementation. *Journal of Nursing Quality Assurance, 1*(2), 31–42.

Deurr, B., & Staats, K. (1988). Quality assurance program evaluation: A view from the unit base. *Journal of Nursing Quality Assurance, 2*(4), 13–16.

Easterbrook, G. (1987, January). The revolution in medicine. *Newsweek*, pp. 40–74.

Fournies, F. (1988). *Why employees don't do what they're supposed to do and what to do about it*. Blue Ridge Summit, PA: TAB Books, Inc. (Liberty House).

Hays, M. (1987). Consumers base quality perceptions on patient relations, staff qualifications. *Modern Healthcare, 17*(5), 33.

Joint Commission on Accreditation of Healthcare Organizations. (1988a). *Examples of monitoring and evaluating in emergency services*. Chicago: Author.

Joint Commission on Accreditation of Healthcare Organizations. (1988b). *Examples of monitoring and evaluating in obstetrics and gynecology*. Chicago: Author.

Joint Commission on Accreditation of Healthcare Organizations. (1988c). *Examples of monitoring and evaluating in special care units*. Chicago: Author.

Joint Commission on Accreditation of Healthcare Organizations. (1989a). Nursing services. In *Joint Commission 1990 Accreditation Manual for Hospitals* (pp. 125–135). Chicago: Author.

Joint Commission on Accreditation of Healthcare Organizations. (1989b). Quality Assurance. In *Joint Commission 1990 Accreditation Manual for Hospitals* (pp. 211–217). Chicago: Author.

Kaye, R. (1988). Quality assurance—a strategy for planned change. In R. Luke, & J. Kruger (Eds.), *Organization and change in health care quality assurance* (pp. 166–167). Rockville, MD: Aspen Publishers.

Lang, N., & Clinton, J. (1984). Assessment of quality of nursing care. *Annual Review of Nursing Research, 2*, 135–163.

Lieske, A. (1985). Standards: The base of a quality assurance program. In C. Meisenheimer (Ed.), *Quality assurance—A complete guide to effective programs* (pp. 45–63). Rockville, MD: Aspen Publishers.

Magin, R., & Pipe, P. (1970). *Analyzing performance problems*. Belmont, CA: Pitman Learning.

Marker, C. (1987). The Marker model: A hierarchy for nursing standards. *Journal of Nursing Quality Assurance, 1*(2), 7–20.

Milton, D. (1988). Challenges of quality assurance evaluation in a practice setting. *Joural of Nursing Quality Assurance, 2*(4), 25–35.

Nadzam, D., & Atkins, M. (1987). The pyramid for quality assurance. *Journal of Nursing Quality Assurance, 2*(1), 13–20.

Naisbitt, J. (1982). *Megatrends*. New York: Warner Books.

Patterson, C. (1989). Standards of patient care: The Joint Commission focus on nursing quality assurance. *Nursing Clinics of North America, 23*(3), 625–638.

Peterson, K. (1988). *The strategic approach to quality service in health care*. Rockville, MD: Aspen Publishers.

Polit, D., & Hungler, B. (1987). *Nursing research—Principles and methods* (3rd ed.). Philadelphia: J.B. Lippincott.

Poster, E., & Pelletier, L. (1988). Part 2: Quantitative and qualitative approaches to nursing program evaluation. *Journal of Nursing Quality Assurance, 2*(4), 63–72.

Poteet, G., & Hodges, L. (1987). The future of nursing. In K. Vestal (Ed.), *Management concepts for the new nurse* (pp. 349–362). Philadelphia: J. B. Lippincott.

Saum, M. (1988). Evaluation: A vital component of the quality assurance program. *Journal of Nursing Quality Assurance, 2*(4), 17–24.

Smeltzer, C. (1988). Evaluating a successful quality assurance program: The process. *Journal of Nursing Quality Assurance, 2*(4), 1–10.

Steiber, S. (1988). How consumers perceive health care policy. *Hospitals, 62*(7), 84.

Watson, C., Bulechek, G., & McCloskey, J. (1987). QAMUR: A quality assurance model using research. *Journal of Nursing Quality Assurance, 2*(1), 21–87.

Westfall, U. (1987). Standards of practice: Nursing values made easy. *Journal of Nursing Quality Assurance, 1*(2), 21–30.

4

Monitoring Practice: A Mental Health Example

Luc R. Pelletier, MSN, RN, CS, Regional Clinical Specialist; Psychiatric Institutes of America, Inc.; Long Beach, California; Former Director, Quality Management, Assistant Hospital Administrator, UCLA Neuropsychiatric Institute and Hospital, Assistant Clinical Professor, UCLA School of Nursing, Los Angeles, California

QUALITY IN MENTAL HEALTH SETTINGS

The process of monitoring and evaluating quality of care in mental health settings is similar to quality assurance (QA) and improvement activities in other health care arenas. The difference lies in the aspects of care and the clinical indicators unique to mental health settings. Principles of quality assurance, quality improvement, and quality control are employed in a systematic, continuous fashion to achieve desired clinical patient outcomes.

The development of standards of measurement in mental health settings has been long in coming. A major difficulty lies in developing indicators that are clinically meaningful for those clinicians providing direct care. This is complicated by the various delivery settings as well as by the varied patient populations served. In mental health settings, clinicians include psychiatrists, neurologists, registered nurses, psychologists, social workers, recreation and occupational therapists, nutritionists, and psychiatric technicians. Another difficulty lies in the attainment of consensus among disciplines as to what is meaningful in the measurement and definition of clinical quality. All mental health programs rely on an interdisciplinary model of treatment. In this type of treatment approach, it is not sufficient to evaluate the efficacy of therapy rendered by the primary therapist (many times a psychiatrist) to determine quality of care. The complex interplay of interdisciplinary treatment by an array of clinicians must also be taken into account. In addition, such administrative concerns as utilization of resources, risk management, and infection control are considered in a comprehensive appraisal of quality.

The author wishes to acknowledge Elizabeth C. Poster, PhD, RN, for her leadership in developing the nursing quality assurance program represented in this chapter.

Who performs this evaluation of quality? In one method, clinicians monitor their own practice. This method poses fragmentation and may leave out critical components of treatment rendered by other clinicians who are part of the patient's multidisciplinary team and who provide interdependent clinical functions. For example, review of the quality and appropriateness of occupational therapy by occupational therapists will not uncover all the factors that may have led to a fall. The fact that the patient had earlier in the day received a sedative for a CT scan may not have been known by the occupational therapist who witnessed a fall that afternoon. Another more comprehensive approach involves reviewing within the context of an interdisciplinary peer review committee as well as coordinating monitoring and evaluation activities under a generic, all-encompassing QA program plan.

Wells and Brooks (1988) concur with this interdisciplinary effort and, in addition, propose the following requirements for implementation of an effective QA effort:

- Develop studies to determine the prevalence of the functional impact of specific patient care problems or psychiatric diagnoses.
- Describe the distribution of care for these problems in various health care settings.
- Link the components of the process of care to salient outcomes.
- Undertake studies to evaluate whether education of providers and patients improves the process or the outcome of care. (p. 59)

McGlynn et al. (1988) have proposed an integrative approach to QA research, "building on principles from efficacy, effectiveness, quality assessment and quality assurance research" (p. 157). Their analytical strategy, however, has found gaps in knowledge. One such gap is the need for short-form diagnostic measures for large-scale studies. Guy and Moore (1982) had attempted to deal with one segment of this problem—that of measuring therapeutic effectiveness in an inpatient setting. Their research culminated in the development of a "Goal Attainment Scale for Psychiatric Inpatients." Their initial challenge was to develop criteria that would cross disciplines since "the different theoretical perspectives of treatment team members produce such diverse opinions that everyone rarely agrees on what measures should be used to assess a patient's progress" (p. 19). They believe they have developed a scale that truly measures patient behaviors represented in state institutions and use these data in their QA activities.

THE *AMH* AND ACUTE PSYCHIATRIC PROGRAMS

The Joint Commission on Accreditation of Healthcare Organizations has come full circle with regard to standards specific to psychiatric programs. After being established in 1951, the Joint Commission developed general hospital standards. Specific standards for long-term facilities were developed in 1966, for the mentally retarded in 1969, for psychiatric inpatient facilities in 1970, and for child and adolescent psychiatric facilities in 1974. A separate standards manual was eventually developed as the *Consolidated Standards Manual for Child, Adolescent, and Adult Psychiatric, Alcoholism, and Drug Abuse Facilities and Facilities Serving the Mentally Retarded/Developmentally Disabled (CSM)*. This manual took the place of an *Accreditation Manual for Hospitals (AMH)* for psychiatric facilities. Community mental health standards were added to the *CSM* in 1987. In 1988, the Joint Commission mandated *AMH* standards for the accreditation of acute psychiatric programs. *CSM* standards continue to be applicable to long-term care and forensic psychiatric facilities.

The transition of acute psychiatric programs from the *CSM* to the *AMH* left voids in certain program components. These voids were to be filled as the Joint Commission further developed the *AMH* manual. An example of filling a void has come with the revised standards in the 1990 *AMH*. These pertain to psychiatric practice in these ways:

- *Child/adolescent standards:* based on the following principles for child/adolescent services: competence and coordination, patient rights, normalization of the environment, family coordination, assessment, treatment, education, monitoring and evaluation, and continuity of care; new standards are spread throughout the *1990 AMH*.
- *Quality Assurance:* a revised required characteristic to focus attention on the need to monitor and evaluate care of specific age groups.

KEY PROGRAM GOALS, FACTORS, AND PROGRAM COMPONENTS

Goals

The goals of any QA program in mental health must include the following:

- to provide a clinical treatment program that produces positive effects and desired clinical outcomes
- to identify and define standards of care through clinical standards and clinical policies and procedures
- to make quality assurance a hospitalwide effort, fostering participation from the chief executive officer on the executive level to the nurse's aide on a unit level

- to identify and correct processes that produce undesired clinical outcomes
- to maintain confidentiality of all proceedings, thereby maintaining the dignity of patients served

Factors

For any QA program to be successful, certain factors must exist. These include

- a commitment from the chief executive officer and adequate resources to conduct a hospitalwide program that includes all clinical services
- a strong QA leader who reports to the chief executive officer or another executive level person
- access to computer resources including personal computer-based programs and mainframe capabilities
- functional interdepartmental relationships, especially between quality assurance and risk management, utilization review, the medical staff, infection control, and all clinical services
- a formalized QA program plan that lists program components as well as responsible parties and reporting deadlines
- a mechanism to reward excellence in the quality of care
- a mechanism to study special populations within an organization (e.g., geropsychiatric patients and children/adolescents).

Program Components

Program components should include mechanisms to review the following:

- medication errors
- unusual occurrence reporting/risk management
  —falls
  —contraband
- high-risk patient profiles
- environmental rounds
- patient satisfaction
- seclusion and restraint
- electroconvulsive therapy review

These components, as a whole, make up a comprehensive quality effort.

General descriptions of these program components follow, with case examples from the UCLA Neuropsychiatric Hospital (UCLA–NPH). The UCLA Neuropsychiatric Institute and Hospital (UCLA–NPI&H), made up of a 209-bed acute care facility and ambulatory care services representing 55,000 outpatient visits annually, is one of the world's most reputable centers for psychiatric and neuroscience care. Inpatient services include eight treatment units addressing the psychiatric, developmental, and neurological needs of children, adolescents, adults, and the aged. Ambulatory care services include 23 specialized clinics serving populations of all developmental levels.

THE QA PROGRAM PLAN

A QA program plan is derived from internal regulators, including the mission and goal statements of the institution and its strategic plan, and external regulators, such as Medicare, MediCal, Title 22 of the Welfare and Institutions Code, and the Joint Commission. The institution's strategic plan should include directives on the maintenance or elevation of the high standard of patient care necessary for teaching, service, and research, while strengthening fiscal performance. In view of cutbacks from Medicare and other third-party payers, staff should continuously respond by using stricter criteria for diagnostic workups, by carefully adjusting staffing patterns to the shifting hospital census, and by employing more effective discharge planning and implementation. With these overall strategies, the quality of patient care services should remain high.

All clinical and environmental departments and services should implement formalized QA activities. These departments/services could include nutrition, ambulatory care, admitting and registration, nursing, medical psychology, social work, rehabilitation, special education (inpatient school), speech, language and audiology services, plant technology and safety services (including maintenance, plant engineering, housekeeping, and laundry handling), and any contracted services. Contract services may include anesthesia, audiology, speech pathology, diagnostic radiology (including nuclear medicine), pastoral services, emergency services, pathology and clinical laboratory, pharmaceutical services, material management, physical therapy, respiratory therapy, podiatry, surgery, dental services, and escort services.

Ongoing monitoring and evaluation activities must be delineated in subplans, and a format for writing these is presented in Exhibit 4-1. Clinical indicators are drawn from clinical aspects of care, representing a variety of structure, process, and outcome measures. Quality is measured by the degree to which various standards or criteria are met. Examples of activities at UCLA–NPH are listed in Exhibit 4-2.

Exhibit 4-1 QA Subplan Format

1. Purpose and Philosophy
   Briefly discuss the purpose or meaning behind the development and implementation of a QA subplan for your department/area/program. Always include a statement to the effect that your plan is developed to make operational the NPH Quality Assurance Program Plan. Add a philosophy statement regarding the uniqueness of your services (i.e., a mission statement).
2. Scope and Goals
   Briefly define the scope of your activities and services (inpatient, outpatient, treatment modalities, diagnoses represented, etc.). Describe the goals of the QA subplan in your department/area/program (e.g., feedback to appropriate personnel to increase effectiveness and timely delivery of services).
3. Structure/Responsible Parties
   What mechanism or structure will you use to implement your QA subplan (e.g., monthly meetings)? State who is assigned the authority to oversee and implement the QA process and who is involved in chairing meetings, preparing reports, etc.
4. Objectives
   Identify what your QA activities are meant to accomplish. Action verbs begin objective statements (e.g., Monitor and evaluate standards of care).
5. Indicators
   This section will be devoted to describing the means by which you carry out QA activities. The outline for this section is

   • Critical Aspects of Care
   • Indicators
   • Standards/Thresholds
   • Data Source
   • Frequency and Method of Study
   • Results/Findings (% Compliance with Standard)
   • Problems Identified
   • Recommended Follow-Up/Time Frame/Responsible Individual
6. Evaluation
   Briefly describe the frequency and methodology you will use to evaluate and modify the appropriateness and efficiency of your QA activities.

Source: Courtesy of UCLA Neuropsychiatric Hospital, Quality Management Department, Los Angeles, CA.

A NOTE ON PROGRAM EVALUATION

Program evaluation is a dynamic, never-ending process of discovering methods to improve effectiveness and efficiency. Evaluation at our institution occurs at every meeting. An annual summary of changes and modifications is part of the annual appraisal. As described previously (Pelletier & Poster, 1988), evaluative

Exhibit 4-2 Department/Service Clinical Indicators

Admission and Registration

- patient registration waiting time
- patient satisfaction survey results
- patient processing efficiency

Adult Ambulatory Care

- rate of accidents/mishaps possibly related to psychotropic medication
- suicide/attempted suicide rate
- evaluation of serum levels with patients receiving maintenance lithium carbonate
- rate of unanticipated rehospitalization

Adult Psychiatry Inpatient Service

- patient-patient assaults
- patient-staff assaults
- transfer to an acute medical-surgical hospital
- AMA discharges

Child Ambulatory Care

- therapy has resulted in reasonable progress toward goals established in treatment plan
- all patient visits documented in medical record
- initial treatment plan developed after evaluation phase

Child Psychiatry Inpatient Service

- appropriate special education plans for MR/DD patients
- linkages to community resources for MR/DD patients
- appropriate behavioral plans for MR/DD patients

Contract Services

- volume indicators for lithium and anticonvulsant
- results of lab tests in progress notes within 24 hours
- rejected specimens as they relate to procedure and personnel
- delay in emergency services
- patient satisfaction with pastoral services
- CT scan and MRI utilization studies
- appropriateness of radiological procedures
- radiology reporting turnaround time
- respiratory therapy Code Blue response time

continues

Exhibit 4-2 continued

Medical Psychology

- timeliness of psychological testing
- appropriateness of psychological testing
- appropriateness of psychotherapy and medical coverage

Medical Records

- inpatient chart completion
- concurrent monitoring results
- clinical pertinence reviews

Nursing

- emergency cart and biomedical equipment checks
- simulated Code Blue drills
- nosocomial infection rates
- quality of Johnson Model–based nursing assessment
- medication administration
- patient outcomes per specified nursing interventions

Nutrition Service

- sanitation and infection control
- accuracy of diet order implementation
- appropriateness of diet order to diagnosis
- identification of patients requiring nutritional intervention

Plant Technology and Safety Program

- preventative maintenance program
- safety, disaster drills, and fire drills
- unusual occurrence reviews

Rehabilitation Services

- individualized assessment and plan
- preventive maintenance of equipment/materials
- falls and injuries during OT/RT

Inpatient School

- quality of individual patient school plans
- pre- and postacademic achievement scores
- follow-up from community resources

Exhibit 4-2 continued

Social Work

- documentation (assessments and progress notes)
- discharge follow-up
- social work clinical pertinence

Speech, Language, and Audiology

- turnaround time from assignment to first assessment
- quality of assessment reports

Source: Courtesy of UCLA Neuropsychiatric Hospital, Quality Management Department, Los Angeles, CA.

phases include formative/process, summative/outcome, and utilization-focused. The steps of an evaluation process include the following:

- Identify program components to be evaluated.
- Describe the methodology to be used.
- Analyze and report the findings.
- Make recommendations to implement corrective action.
- Evaluate the impact of corrective action.

Of course, both qualitative and quantitative methods can be used in determining the significance of findings (Poster & Pelletier, 1988). "Assigning numerical meaning to results by use of quantitative methods reveals only a part of any human picture. With the addition of qualitative approaches, the picture becomes whole and meaningful to decision makers. This need for a broader picture is especially true in Nursing QA where human responses are critical factors of concern" (p. 71).

PROGRAM COMPONENTS AND CLINICAL EXAMPLES

The program components of medication errors, unusual occurrence reporting/ risk management, environmental rounds, seclusion and restraint audits, electroconvulsive therapy reviews, and patient satisfaction will be discussed in detail below. The final focus is on nursing quality assurance in mental health.

Medication Errors

Medication errors are tracked for various reasons. Overall, it is necessary to determine why errors are being made and by whom. These data are useful for clinical nurse managers in determining staff education needs as well as in changing the physical plant or the medication administration processes or policies.

Medication errors account for approximately 35 percent of all incidents at UCLA–NPH. The number of unusual occurrences referred to the Nursing QA Committee rose from 14 during fiscal year 1987–88 to 56 in fiscal year 1988–89. The medication error rate remains essentially stable from year to year, at 0.0014.

The highest reporting area is a geropsychiatric unit, followed by a general adult psychiatry unit and a neurology unit. A study was done by Pelletier and Poster (1988) to evaluate the error rates of units that used a functional medication administration system ("medication nurse") versus those that used a primary medication administration system (primary nurses dispensing medications for their own patients). A major finding showed that the error rate was less on units implementing the primary method of medication administration. Further, the overall medication error rate was found to be lower than other previously published medication error rates.

Unusual Occurrence Reporting System/Risk Management

Unusual occurrence (UO) reporting can serve two purposes, that of a quality tool and that of a risk management tool. The UO is completed whenever a clinical or environmental incident occurs that is out of the ordinary. Examples of such incidents should include

- falls, injuries
- skin integrity impairment that occurred previous to hospitalization or during the course of treatment
- suicides, suicide attempts, and self-inflicted injuries
- patient-patient assaults, patient-staff assaults
- medication errors

The flow of information for the UCLA–NPH program is shown in Figure 4-1.

A Risk Management Subcommittee was formed to review those indicators that pose actual and/or potential high risk for claims against the hospital. The subcommittee is concerned with protecting the assets of the organization by reducing the risks of injury associated with being a patient at the NPH. The purposes of the subcommittee's work are to prevent future claims and to provide the QA Commit-

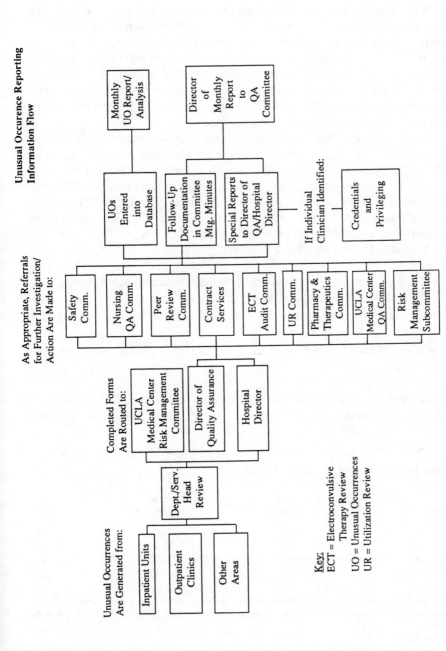

Figure 4-1 Unusual Occurrence Reporting Information Flow. *Source:* Courtesy of UCLA Neuropsychiatric Hospital, Quality Management Department, Los Angeles, CA.

tee with program development strategies that are preventive in nature. The subcommittee reviews data from many sources, including current claims analysis, patient complaints and comments, environmental rounds data, unusual occurrence reports, Safety Committee minutes, and reports from the NPH ombudsperson.

An analysis of 1988–89 fiscal year data is presented in Tables 4-1 and 4-2. In general, the reporting system continues to run smoothly in inpatient areas. Slowly, the ambulatory care areas have adopted the UO as a QA measurement tool. Efforts to educate personnel in those areas will continue.

The Risk Management Subcommittee developed and implemented the following projects: a fall study, a contraband study, and a high-risk patient identification system. The fall study involved an analysis of 500 falls within the past five years. The data for this survey are currently being compiled and prepared for publication. The contraband study was designed to review contraband incidents. (*Contraband* is defined as any potentially harmful object that a patient knowingly brings to the hospital—e.g., a knife, prescription medications, illegal drugs.) The results of the study pointed to these significant findings.

- Patients labeled with major affective disorders are more likely to bring in contraband than are those in other diagnostic categories.
- Contraband is more likely to be confiscated on admission than after a pass or visit.
- No incidents of contraband confiscation resulted in serious patient outcomes (Pelletier, Poster, & Kay, 1990).

The subcommittee also has been developing a high-risk patient identification system. This system involves retrieving historical incident information on patients

---

Table 4-1 Unusual Occurrence Rate by Year

Year	Number of Reported UOs	Number of Patient Days*	Rate
1985–86	1,361	41,023	.03
1986–87	1,248	39,118	.03
1987–88	1,150	36,961	.03
1988–89	1,051	34,192	.03

*Patient days are for inpatients since this is the area most responsive to UO reporting. If patient days also included total outpatient visits, the rates would be 1985–86 (.025); 1986–87 (.02); 1987–88 (.02); 1988–89 (.02).

Source: Courtesy of UCLA Neuropsychiatric Hospital, Quality Management Department, Los Angeles, CA.

Table 4-2 Unusual Occurrences by Type and Frequency

Type*	Number Reported 87–88	Number Reported 88–89	Percentage of Total 87–88 (N = 1,150)	Percentage of Total 88–89 (N = 1,051)	Percentage of Change
Medication error	368	406	32.00	38.62	+6.62
Falls (from bed, getting in/out of bed, during seizure, other than above)	149	156	12.95	14.84	+1.89
Injuries (sustained during seizure, while ambulatory, while being restrained, from fallen or thrown object)	114	79	9.91	7.51	−2.4
Self-inflicted injury	66	64	5.73	6.08	+0.35
Accident during OT/RT	60	41	5.21	3.90	−1.31

*Represented are the five most frequently reported events for FY 1987–1988 compared with FY 1988–89 data. The data are taken from the Unusual Occurrence Program in the Quality Assurance Department. It is important to mention that 94 incidents (8.94 percent) were coded as "Other." This is compared to last year's figure of 145 (12.87 percent) ranked as "Other." Our assumption that the revision of UO types may decrease the number of "Other" categorizations may be correct.

Source: Courtesy of UCLA Neuropsychiatric Hospital, Quality Management Department, Los Angeles, CA.

admitted to the hospital from a computer program. This information is then routed to the assigned clinician and primary nurse for inclusion in the data base and treatment plan. For example, if a patient's incident history reveals several falls during a prior hospitalization on a geropsychiatric unit, this patient could be considered high risk for future falls and/or injuries during this hospitalization. Clinicians would be given this information to prepare treatment plans for potential falls and injuries. UCLA–NPH implemented this program in January 1990.

Environmental Rounds

Under recent guidelines developed by the Joint Commission, clinical safety has become a focus of interest. Not only are hospitals encouraged to identify hazards, but also they must establish a preventive program that identifies potential hazards and a mechanism to correct such potential problems. Such a formal preventive mechanism exists at UCLA–NPH.

The Environmental Rounds Program was developed to enhance the monitoring and evaluation activities relating to the physical plant and clinical safety. A general purpose of the rounds is to ensure compliance with internal policies and procedures as well as with the policies and procedures of external regulatory agencies such as the Joint Commission, Title 22, and Medicare/MediCal. A team of executive-level managers meets monthly to survey selected areas in the hospital and ambulatory care facility. Each hospital and ambulatory care area is surveyed twice a year. The survey team uses an environmental rounds checklist, which lists criteria to be evaluated during the rounds. Unit personnel are invited to "round" with the surveyors and to correct problems immediately as they are found. The environmental rounds information flow is presented in Figure 4-2; examples of environmental rounds criteria are listed in Exhibit 4-3.

Discharge Indicators/Peer Review

Multidisciplinary peer review committees afford a hospital the opportunity to review individual cases comprehensively since members of the treatment team are represented.

Peer review committees have been formed in all clinical divisions at UCLA–NPH. Each committee is chaired by a physician, and members include representatives from the professional staff (registered nurses, psychologists, social workers). Agendas include the review of unusual occurrences referred to the committee, patient satisfaction questionnaire responses that warrant investigation, and discharge indicator reviews. All clinical divisions review the following discharge indicators monthly:

- length of stay (adult >30, child >80, neurology >10)
- against medical advice
- readmission within 15 or 30 days
- discharge to an acute medical-surgical hospital
- death
- Code Blue
- transfusion

Computer-generated lists of indicators are reviewed by the director of quality assurance, and assignments are made to peer review committee members. These committee members then review medical records using predetermined review criteria and report their findings in the peer review committee's minutes. Peer review information on individual clinicians is routed to a credentials and privileging file in the medical staff office, which assures the link between clinical review findings and the reappointment process. Written and verbal reports are made monthly before the peer review committees. Examples of review criteria are listed in Exhibit 4-4.

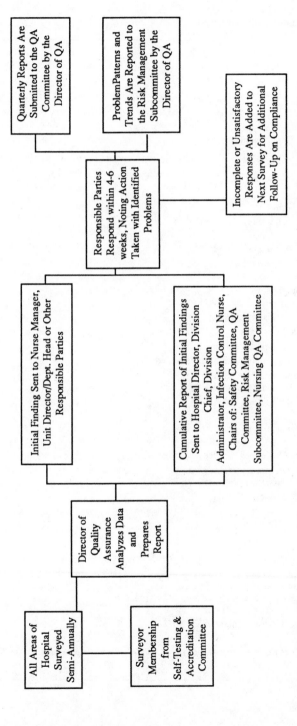

Figure 4-2 Environmental Rounds Information Flow. *Source:* Courtesy of UCLA Neuropsychiatric Hospital, Quality Management Department, Los Angeles, CA.

Exhibit 4-3 Environmental Rounds Criteria

1. **Item**
   - Beds
   Criteria
   - Functional
   - Safe
   - Age and type appropriate
   Responsible Department/Service
   - Facilities & Services, Nursing
2. **Item**
   - Emergency equipment
   Criteria
   - Emergency drugs
   - EKG/defibrillator/suction/oxygen
   - Crash cart functional
   Responsible Department/Service
   - Nursing, contract services
3. **Item**
   - Medications/supplies
   Criteria
   - Internals/externals separate
   - Open medications dated
   - Medications current (not expired)
   - Metric and weight conversion charts posted
   - Poison control telephone number posted
   Responsible Department/Service
   - Nursing
4. **Item**
   - Patient's personal appliances
   Criteria
   - Checked by Facilities & Services
   - Appliances not in use unless tagged
   Responsible Department/Service
   - Facilities & Services, Nursing
5. **Item**
   - Earthquake Preparedness
   Criteria
   - Present as needed:
     —Seismic monitoring
     —Flashlights/batteries
     —Transistor radio/batteries
     —Staff attendance at earthquake preparedness classes
   Responsible Department/Service
   - Facilities & Services, Unit/Division Staff

Source: Courtesy of UCLA Neuropsychiatric Hospital, Quality Management Department, Los Angeles, CA.

Exhibit 4-4 Discharge Indicator Review Criteria

Length of Stay (LOS)

- Was LOS due to
  —a placement problem?
  —a disposition problem?
  —a legal problem?
  —an unanticipated medical problem?
- Were weekly progress notes regarding discharge planning present?

Against Medical Advice (AMA)

- Could the AMA discharge reasonably have been anticipated or prevented?
- Did the patient exhibit symptoms that would have warranted a 72-hold?
- Were the patient's complaints legitimate and not adequately dealt with prior to discharge?
- If there was a complaint, was it due to inadequate or substandard care?

Readmission

- Why was the patient readmitted?
- Was the patient's previous discharge premature, given the severity of illness?
- Is there a relationship between the reason for readmission and the patient's previous hospitalization?
- Is the readmission due to a deficiency in discharge planning?

Source: Courtesy of UCLA Neuropsychiatric Hospital, Quality Management Department, Los Angeles, CA.

The adult division generated the most discharge indicators, followed by the child division and then neurology. From an analysis of the data, it was decided that length of stay triggers would be fine-tuned. For example, in adult psychiatry, some diagnoses typically required more than 30 days of hospitalization. Therefore, patients who were diagnosed with obsessive-compulsive disorder would be triggered if their length of stay was greater than 60 days; those patients who had undergone electroconvulsive therapy would be triggered if they stayed longer than 50 days. In child psychiatry, those patients with anorexia nervosa would be triggered only if they stayed longer than 130 days. Significant accomplishments of the peer review committees included revision of Code Blue criteria to include autopsy information, development of clinical monitoring criteria in neurology, and initiation of medical record clinical pertinence reviews.

Seclusion and Restraint Audits

Since seclusion and restraint procedures limit an individual's freedom, and since strict guidelines govern such denials of rights, these procedures must be monitored closely. Many hospitals have retrospective reviews of records to determine adherence to policies and procedures. Recently, UCLA–NPH moved away from retrospective reviews to more timely concurrent reviews of medical records.

Originally, seclusion and restraint audits had been part of the nightly nurse audit conducted on each nursing unit. These reviews were supplemented by the QA department's semiannual retrospective medical record audits. Recently, because clinicians need more timely information, the QA department has taken on the responsibility of reviewing seclusion and restraint incidents concurrently and providing feedback to clinicians regarding deficiencies in policy requirements or procedures. The seclusion and restraint review criteria are illustrated in Exhibit 4-5.

The seclusion rate for fiscal year 1988–89 was .016. The rate for restraint for the same period was .006. The calculation used for seclusion and restraint rates is

Number of incidents ÷ number of patient days for the year

These annual data are used by risk management and each clinical division to analyze utilization.

Electroconvulsive Therapy Review

Although procedures for electroconvulsive therapy (ECT) have been perfected over the years, this treatment continues to be considered high risk in some populations. Since the procedure involves anesthesia and other support services, monitoring and evaluation are critical.

The medical records audits of patients who undergo ECT at UCLA–NPH are reviewed concurrently by the Medical Records department. Further, an ECT Review Committee meets quarterly to review utilization as required by state and county regulations. The committee consists of six members, two of whom must be physicians knowledgeable about ECT. An ECT Consultant Panel serves to meet California Administrative Code requirements for purposes of independent review and consultation. Examples of audit criteria for voluntary and involuntary ECT cases are presented in Exhibit 4-6.

Patient Satisfaction

In today's health climate, a happy customer (patient) is a customer who may return for services at a later date. A disgruntled customer, on the other hand, won't

Exhibit 4-5 Quality Assurance–Concurrent Review Behavioral Seclusion and Restraint Standards

Part IA		Physician's Orders					
Policy 2005 Reference	*Procedure 2005.1 Reference*	*Criteria*	*Met*	*Not Met*	*N/A*	*Comments*	*Follow-Up*
3	1.1	A written order for Behavior Restraint/Seclusion is in Doctor's orders (within 1 hour of initial use of Seclusion/Restraint)					
4.1	1.1.1	Order states reason for Restraint/Seclusion					
4.2 5.3.3	1.1.2 1.2	Order is time limited and does not exceed 24 hours					
4.3	1.1.3	PRN order not valid					
5		In an emergency: Verbal order is written by clinically privileged RN on Doctor's Order Sheet					
5.3.2	1.4	Verbal order is countersigned by MD within 12 hours of giving verbal order; countersignature is dated and timed					
8	1.3	If S/R is utilized *continuously* for a period of greater than 24 hours, a new order is written and countersigned by the Unit Director or designee					

continues

Exhibit 4-5 continued

Part IB — Progress Notes—Physician

Policy Reference	Procedure Reference	Criteria	Met	Not Met	N/A	Comments	Follow-Up
5.4	1.1.5	Progress Note documents the rationale for the use of Behavioral Restraint					
4.4 5.5	1.1.4	Progress Note states why less restrictive interventions were ineffective					
11	2.1.1	Unusual frequency or pattern of use addressed					

Part IIA — Progress Notes—Nursing

Policy Reference	Procedure Reference	Criteria	Met	Not Met	N/A	Comments	Follow-Up
	6.1.1	In an emergency, a Progress Note is written by an RN					
5.4		Progress Note documents clinical assessment of need for Behavioral Restraint					
5.5		Progress Note states why less restrictive interventions were ineffective					
	6.1.2	When an Unusual Occurrence happens during the time the patient is in Behavioral Restraint or Seclusion, the staff member observing the incident records the information					
	6.1.3	When a patient is placed in Behavioral Restraint or Seclusion for the first time, the registered nurse assigned to the patient for the given shift records the information					
	6.1.4	A minimum of one Progress Note is written by an RN for each shift in which Behavioral Seclusion/Restraint occurs					

Part IIB	Restraint/Seclusion Record (Form #1-084)					
Policy Procedure Code	Criteria	Met	Not Met	N/A	Comments	Follow-Up
6.2.1	Date and time placed in Seclusion/Restraint					
6.2.2	Initial of staff completing the patient environment checks for potentially dangerous articles					
6.2.3	Rationale/reason for Restraint/Seclusion					
6.2.4	Type of R/S being used (i.e., #1 Seclusion, #2 Restraint) and extremities involved					
6.2.5	Criteria for discontinuance are in behavioral terms					
6.1 5.3	Clock hour patient was checked at a minimum of 15-minute intervals (and more frequently if indicated by patient's condition)					
6.2.7	Patient's response to Seclusion/Restraint care given as it relates to nutrition, fluids, exercise, elimination, support, personal hygiene (behaviorally defined)					
6.2.8	Time of rotation of restraints is recorded					
4.10.2	Restraints released every 2 hours for a minimum of five minutes; if contradicted, remove one extremity at a time for five minutes					
6.2.9	Time patient is removed from Seclusion/Restraint, patient's response, staff signature					
6.2.10	Staff initials and writes signature that includes first initial, last name, and classification					

Comments:

Source: Courtesy of UCLA Neuropsychiatric Hospital, Quality Management Department, Los Angeles, CA.

Exhibit 4-6 ECT Audit Criteria

- Adequate documentation is in the medical record, signed by the treatment attending physicians,
  —of the reason for the procedure
  —that all reasonable treatment modalities were considered
  —that treatment was definitely indicated and was the least drastic alternative available at the time
- Properly completed, executed, and witnessed informed ECT and anesthesiology consents are filed in the medical record.
- Consultation is obtained for patients receiving >15 ECT treatments within 30 days or >30 ECT treatments within a one-year period.
- Complications, if any, are addressed in the progress or procedure note.
- The presence or absence of postanesthesia complications is documented in the medical record.

Source: Courtesy of UCLA Neuropsychiatric Hospital, Quality Management Department, Los Angeles, CA.

---

return. As Marker (1989) puts it, "Pleased patients seldom sue." Basic marketing techniques used in the business sector tell us that we must be acutely aware of the customers' point of view and their satisfaction with services rendered. This industrial premise is currently flowing into the health care sector, as quality improvement focuses on customer needs and their resultant satisfaction with services and products. Prehn (1989) points out that "it is only fair and democratic that patients, whose lives may be deeply influenced by health care decisions, should have a voice in making those decisions" (p. 74).

For satisfaction to be measured, you must first know what the patient expects. Many times, the negative comments we have reviewed have resulted from unfulfilled or misunderstood expectations of service. "I thought I would have a private room," "I thought I could bring in my television and VCR," "Someone told me I'd see the doctor every day for 2 hours," and "My nurse didn't talk to me enough" are remarks from dissatisfied customers. When reviewing such remarks, hospital managers have to wonder about what was covered during the admission interview when such unrealistic expectations should have been discussed. Hospital staff must balance patient expectations with milieu safety by using teaching and negotiation to explain realistic expectations and goals.

The patient satisfaction survey system at UCLA–NPH was developed to meet these goals.

- All clients will be given the opportunity to give feedback about their hospital/clinic experience in the form of a patient satisfaction questionnaire.

- Any client who requests feedback about an issue will be contacted by a hospital manager.

The information flow regarding patient satisfaction is illustrated in Figure 4-3. Examples from the 53-item structured inpatient questionnaire format include the following:

- If you were not admitted within a reasonable length of time, was the delay caused by:
  a. no delay
  b. missing paperwork
  c. room was not ready
  d. other delay—please explain
  e. reason was not explained to me
- Were the nurses helpful in explaining procedures and answering questions?
- Rate the nursing staff's concern for you as a person as well as a patient.
- Did you feel that your nurses were skilled and capable?
- Overall, how would you rate nursing services?
- Who was your primary nurse?
- Were medications and medication side effects clearly explained to you?

Separate formats have been developed for child, adult, and neurology ambulatory care services. Following are examples from an adult ten-item questionnaire:

- How would you rate the manner in which the therapist treats you?
- How would you rate our fee structure and billing procedures?
- As a result of your treatment, how would you rate your present condition?
- How likely is it that you would refer a friend or relative to NPH?

Although the patient satisfaction survey system is the primary source of patient feedback about UCLA–NPH services, the patient is also informed about the services of the hospital ombudsperson. The ombudsperson's role is to gather any information from a patient/family member and investigate the situation, many times including established hospitalwide committees such as the Peer Review and Nursing QA committees.

The current return rate of patient satisfaction questionnaires is 16.7 percent. The majority of the responses have been in the "good" to "fair" categories (possible responses include excellent, good, fair, poor, and not applicable). The areas of discharge planning and outpatient follow-up were the most significant problem areas, as identified by patients who responded to the questionnaire, which

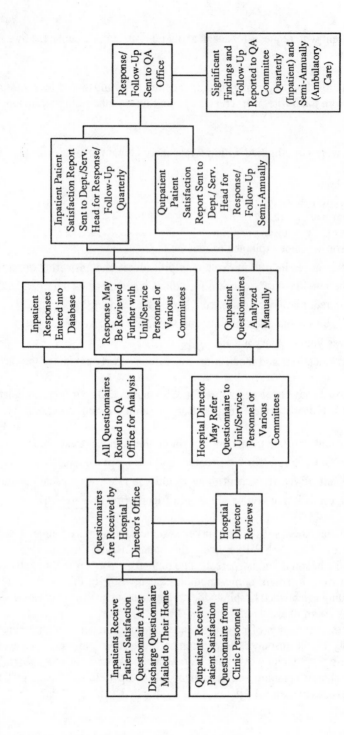

Figure 4-3 Patient Satisfaction Information Flow. *Source:* Courtesy of UCLA Neuropsychiatric Hospital, Quality Management Department, Los Angeles, CA.

was mailed one week after discharge. Whereas findings were previously generated annually for review, we have moved to a quarterly analysis and reporting schedule. Efforts have been made to increase the response rate (e.g., by having social workers pass out the questionnaire at discharge). Some units are currently yielding response rates as high as 36 percent. We are now investigating the feasibility of telephone interviews after discharge to increase the number of patient satisfaction responses. We will be securing advice from our legal counsel in order to protect the confidentiality of patients and their communications to us.

NURSING QUALITY ASSURANCE IN MENTAL HEALTH

A formalized nursing QA program is critical to any hospital's success. Since nurses are with patients longer than any other professional is, they are armed with much information about the processes of care and when these processes break down. Their input is crucial to understanding the special problems that are encountered on a psychiatric unit.

The Nursing Quality Assurance Committee (NQAC), chaired by the director of nursing education and research, is the pivotal organizing structure for nursing QA activities at UCLA–NPH. The purpose of the committee (which serves as the operational unit of the Nursing QA Program) is to monitor and evaluate the quality and effectiveness of nursing care based on accepted standards of nursing practice. The NQAC provides a feedback mechanism to all nursing staff regarding the current level of nursing care, the relevancy of established nursing standards, and the identification and resolution of patient care problems.

The patient care services reviewed through the NQAC include

* nursing process
* special treatment procedures
* medication administration
* unusual occurrences

Data sources used to identify actual and potential nursing care problems include

* nurses' observations through medical record documentation
* staff concerns
* patient/family feedback
* various UCLA–NPH committee reports
* policies and procedures
* concurrent, retrospective, and outcome reviews

- reports from external regulatory agencies/facilities
- unusual occurrence reports
- current research literature and clinical practice

Communication among all parties involved in nursing QA activities is facilitated by

- committee minutes and annual reports
- Nursing QA Master Plan
- special studies (see Exhibit 4-7)
- nursing care indicators (see Table 4-3)
- Quality Assurance Reporting Form (see Exhibit 4-8)

Significant outcomes of QA efforts are found throughout the eight inpatient clinical units.

- Inservice education classes were given to adolescent unit nursing staff on reading tuberculin skin tests (PPDs); this training resulted in a decreased lag time between the physician's order for the PPD and its administration/reading.
- Feedback was given to nursing staff on units that had studied (1) documentation of patient teaching regarding medications and their side effects and (2) documentation of vital signs; compliance with standards increased significantly as these areas continued to be monitored and evaluated.
- The nosocomial infection rate for fiscal year 1988–89 was 4.9 percent, with a range of 1.9 to 6.1 percent.
- Classes on universal precautions were held by the nurse epidemiologist, and a follow-up study was conducted regarding hand-washing practices and basic infection control techniques.
- Monthly monitoring of patient falls on a geropsychiatric unit resulted in the identification of multiple fallers and a study on patient outcome.
- Special studies included IV, Admission Assessment Study, Staff Satisfaction/Work Environment, Phlebitis Follow-Up, Patient Satisfaction, Ativan/Xanax Investigation, Seizure Evaluation, and Hand-Washing Study. Outcomes of these studies resulted in inservice classes, changes in unit documentation, development of new policies and procedures, and individual counseling of staff to improve performance.

Over the past few months, the NQAC has endeavored to develop more outcome-oriented indicators. This has resulted in a focus on patient outcomes in the

Exhibit 4-7 Nursing QA Report

Date Study Initiated _____

Date Study Completed _____

Date NQAC Review of Findings _____

Date Findings Reported to Staff _____

Nursing Q.A. Committee Item # _____

Nursing Unit _____

Total Hours of Data Collection _____

Total Cost _____

Data Collector(s) _____

IDENTIFIED PROBLEM OR STANDARD BEING MONITORED:

Identified by _____

Date _____

METHODOLOGY (Information Collection Process):

continues

Exhibit 4-7 continued

FINDINGS:

RECOMMENDATIONS/CORRECTIVE ACTION TAKEN:

Person Responsible _____

Date _____

PLAN FOR EVALUATION OF IMPACT OF CORRECTIVE ACTION(S):

Time Frame _____

Source: Courtesy of UCLA Neuropsychiatric Hospital, Nursing Department, Los Angeles, CA.

Table 4-3 Quality Assurance Monitoring of Nursing Care Indicators

Indicators	Data Sources	Standard/Threshold	Frequency of Monitor
Medication Administration	Unusual Occurrence Reports Medication Administration Record Pharmacy data: # Doses of Medication by Unit	Medication error rates >1%	Daily review of UO reports Monthly summaries analyzed for trends and patterns
Infection Rates	Infection Control Reports Medical Record Laboratory Reports	Nosocomial infection rate of zero	Daily review of IC reports Monthly summary reports
Evacuation/Fire Drills	Fire Drill Log (Nursing Office)	Four times a year—per shift, per unit	Quarterly
Mock Code Drills	Simulated CPR Audit Forms	Once per year—per shift, per unit	Annually
Staff Satisfaction	Staff Satisfaction Questionnaire		Annually
Patient/Family Satisfaction	Discharge Patient Satisfaction Questionnaire Responses		Following discharge of all inpatients
Predicted Patient Outcomes	Medical Record	80% of predicted outcomes are achieved	Concurrent review
Outcome of Patient Falls	Unusual Occurrence Reports	100% of patient falls have nonconsequential outcomes	Concurrent review Monthly report
Medication Incident Outcomes	Medical Record Unusual Occurrence Reports	100% of medication errors have nonconsequential outcomes	Retrospective or concurrent review Monthly report

Source: Courtesy of UCLA Neuropsychiatric Hospital, Nursing Department, Los Angeles, CA.

Exhibit 4-8 Quality Assurance Monthly Monitor Summary

SUBMITTED FROM: _____   SUBMITTED TO: _____

(department)

NAME: _____

MONTH/YEAR: _____

Indicator	Standard/Threshold	Data Source	Frequency & Method	Results/Findings/ Rating*	Problems Identified	Recommended Follow-Up & Responsible Staff

COMMENTS:

*Please *rate* each monitoring activity as follows: 1. substantial compliance, 2. significant compliance, 3. partial compliance, 4. minimal compliance, 5. noncompliance, 6. N/A (Not Applicable) (to be used with volume indicators only).

Report is due on third Monday of the month (for previous month's activities). Please send copy to Director of Quality Assurance and save copy for your records. Copy retained for one year in QA Office.

Source: Courtesy of UCLA Neuropsychiatric Hospital, Quality Management Department, Los Angeles, CA.

following areas: aggressive-protective subsystem (of the Johnson Behavioral System Model), seclusion and restraint, falls, medication knowledge, eating disorders, electroconvulsive therapy, and clinical safety.

CONCLUSION

Quality assurance activities in mental health are effective to the extent that the issues identified and addressed are meaningful to a variety of mental health clinicians. The challenge for chief executive officers and directors of quality assurance is to involve the full cadre of mental health professionals and administrators in the planning and execution of a comprehensive QA program. When the task is clear and responsible parties are identified, a systematic flow of information is established, which meets internal and external regulatory reviews.

Quality assurance processes have a way of changing practice—but only when the development of standards and the evaluation of treatment outcomes are shared hospital responsibilities.

BIBLIOGRAPHY

Cahn, C., & Richman, A. (1985). Quality assurance in psychiatry. *Canadian Journal of Psychiatry,* *3*(2), 148–152.

Ehrhart, K. (1989). Implementing the 10-step QA model in a state psychiatric multi-hospital system. *Journal of Quality Assurance,* 12–13 + .

Evans, C.L.S., & Lewis, S.K. (1985). *Nursing administration of psychiatric–mental health care.* Rockville, MD: Aspen Publishers.

Fauman, M.A. (1989). Quality assurance monitoring in psychiatry. *American Journal of Psychiatry,* *146*(9), 1121–1130.

Fleming, J.L. (1989). Business values and quality in psychiatric hospital treatment. *Psychiatric Hospital,* *20*(3), 115–118.

Graham, J. (1987, February). Quality gets a closer look. *Modern Healthcare,* pp. 20–31.

Guy, M.E., & Moore, L.S. (1982). The goal attainment scale for psychiatric inpatients. *Quality Review Bulletin,* 19–29.

Hadley, T.R., & McGurrin, M.C. (1988). Accreditation, certification, and the quality of care in psychiatric hospitals. *Hospital and Community Psychiatry,* *39*(7), 739–742.

Joint Commission on Accreditation of Healthcare Organizations. (1987). *Consolidated standards manual for child, adolescent, and adult psychiatric, alcoholism, and drug abuse facilities and facilities serving the mentally retarded/developmentally disabled.* Chicago: Author.

Joint Commission on Accreditation of Healthcare Organizations. (1990). *1990 accreditation manual for hospitals.* Chicago: Author.

Kibbee, P., & Lilly, G. (1989). Outcome-oriented documentation in a psychiatric facility. *Journal of Quality Assurance,* 16–21.

McGlynn, E.A., Norquist, G.S., Wells, K.B., Sullivan, G., & Liberman, R.P. (1988). Quality of care research in mental health: Responding to the challenge. *Inquiry,* *25*, 157–170.

Maciorowski, L.F., Munro, B.H., Dietrick-Gallagher, M., McNew, C.D., Sheppard. Hirikel, E., Wanick, C., & Ragan, P.A. (1988). A review of the patient fall data. *Journal of Nursing Quality Assurance, 3*(1), 18–27.

Marker, J. (1989). Integrating patient satisfaction into your QA/RM program—Or pleased patients seldom sue. *Journal of Quality Assurance,* 8–10 +.

Morse, J.M., & Morse, R.M. (1988). Calculating fall rates: Methodological concerns. *Quality Review Bulletin,* 369–371.

Morse, J.M., Prowse, M.D., Morrow, N., & Federspeil, G. (1985). A retrospective analysis of patient falls. *Canadian Journal of Public Health, 76,* 116–118.

Pelletier, L.R., & Poster, E.C. (1988). Part I: An overview of evaluation methodology for nursing quality assurance programs. *Journal of Nursing Quality Assurance, 2*(4), 55–61.

Pelletier, L.R., Poster, E.C., & Kay, I.C. (1990). Contraband: The hidden risk. *Quality Review Bulletin, 16*(1), 9–14.

Poster, E.C., & Pelletier, L.R. (1988). Primary versus functional medication administration: Monitoring and evaluating medication error rates. *Journal of Nursing Quality Assurance, 2*(2), 68–76.

Poster, E.C., & Pelletier, L.R. (1988). Part II: Quantitative and qualitative approaches to nursing quality assurance program evaluation. *Journal of Nursing Quality Assurance, 2*(4), 63–72.

Prehn, R.A. (1989). Determining the validity of patient perceptions of quality care. *Quality Review Bulletin,* 74–76.

Silverman, W.H. (1988). Patient care monitoring review at a psychiatric hospital for adolescents. *Quality Review Bulletin,* 307–310.

Smeltzer, C.H., Hirishaw, A.S., & Feltman, B. (1987). The benefits of staff nurse involvement in monitoring the quality of patient care. *Journal of Nursing Quality Assurance, 1*(3), 1–7.

Stevenson, J.F., Beattie, M.C., Alves, R.R., Longabaugh, R., & Ayers, T. (1988). An outcome monitoring system for psychiatric inpatient care. *Quality Review Bulletin,* 326–331.

Stricker, G., & Rodriguez, A.R. (Eds.). (1988). *Handbook of quality assurance in mental health.* New York: Plenum.

Tischler, G.L., & Astrachan, B. (1982). *Quality assurance in mental health: Peer and utilization review.* Rockville, MD: U.S. Department of Health and Human Services.

Wells, K.B., & Brooks, R.H. (1988). Historical trends in quality assurance for mental health services. In G. Stricker & A.R. Rodriguez (Eds.), *Handbook of quality assurance in mental health.* New York: Plenum, p. 39.

5

Monitoring Practice: A Critical Care Example

Ann Libka Hendrich, MSN, RN, Clinical Research Nurse, Medical Research/ Critical Care, Methodist Hospital of Indiana Inc., Indianapolis, Indiana

THE CRITICAL CARE ENVIRONMENT

By definition, the profession of critical care nursing acts "to deal with human responses to life threatening problems" (Sanford & Disch, 1989). Intensive care or critical care can reflect many different types of specialized care units where seriously ill patients receive medical and nursing care. Terms such as *coronary, neurological, surgical, medical, pediatric,* and *pulmonary* are frequently applied to denote even more specific areas of critical care. In these units, where critically ill patients are at high risk for additional complications from their illnesses, their nursing care requires frequent nursing assessments, nursing and medical interventions, and collaborative approaches to decision making in order to maintain optimal patient outcomes.

The role of nurses who practice in critical care units is an example of the "expanded role," in that they deal with a particular environment and highly specialized equipment, and they are required to make rapid decisions based on nursing assessments and interventions that often have a direct effect on patient outcomes. These interventions may be independent, dependent, or interdependent and act to stabilize, prevent complications, and promote optimal outcomes. Each type of nursing intervention is characterized by the level of the nurse's involvement as a decision maker. *Dependent interventions* are used with those problems that are the direct responsibility of the physician, who then designates specific interventions for the nurse. Collaborative efforts by physicians or other allied health professionals in prescribing and treating patient problems or clinical conditions are *interdependent interventions*. *Independent interventions* occur when the

The author wishes to acknowledge the Methodist Hospital of Indiana's Medical Research and the Critical Care departments for their support and contributions.

nurse has direct responsibility for preventing, reducing, or alleviating the problem (Carpenito, 1983).

In addition to the patient, the critical care nurse also cares for the family of the critically ill patient. Bozett and Gibbons (1983) identified "information gathering" about the patient as a strategy that facilitates adaptation and coping during the state of crisis. Because the CCN is often a constant at the bedside, he or she is the most dependable informational source for the critically ill patient's family. Meeting these informational needs may help to reduce stress, maintain homeostasis, and assist the family in adapting to the crisis.

The scope, then, of critical care nursing practice can be defined and measured by the relationship between the critical care nurse, the critically ill patient, and the critical care environment. The quality of nursing care can be measured and defined by monitoring aspects of each of the above three elements. As the critical care system becomes more complex, with additional advanced technology being used in a cost-conscious environment, the measurement of these attributes within the domains of quality, appropriateness, and patient outcome will become vital for the management of all critical care units.

REVIEW OF THE LITERATURE

The traditional approach to quality assurance (QA), in which centralized retrospective audits were the sole mechanism for the evaluation of patient care, has given way to more progressive and innovative approaches in most health care facilities. Audits have been replaced by such innovations as nursing rounds, peer review, group problem solving by task forces, measurement tool development, and questionnaires designed to measure patient education (Gawlinski, 1982).

It is evident that quality assurance has undergone rapid changes since its introduction into nursing practice in the mid-1970s. These changes are apparent in the few articles written about quality assurance in critical care settings, and the approaches may vary. However, certain aspects and needs of quality assurance in critical care or intensive care units remain congruent in the literature. At least two consistent ideas are present.

First, there is a need for a unit-based approach, as described by Schroeder and Maibusch (1984) and by Pinkerton and Schroeder (1988). Such an approach brings QA functions to the unit level with a unit policy and/or QA plan that clearly delineates the methods by which nursing practice will be evaluated. Second, there is a recognized need to consistently and objectively measure quality through a nursing standard. Gawlinski discussed the notion that Critical Care Standards, as defined by the American Association of Critical Care Nurses (AACN), could be used in two ways: (1) to evaluate job performance and (2) to evaluate nursing care practices. Specifically, there is an urgent need to integrate these standards of care into the unit QA program in order to define strengths and areas that need improvement in the critical care unit.

Rowe and Jackson (1989) described the value of a multidisciplinary concurrent approach to quality assurance, necessary because of the increasingly complex patient care setting. A critical care quality assurance monitor was used to track medical complications, while reviewing nursing care. Incorporated into the QA process, this concurrent audit tool replaced the ineffective retrospective report, which included only demographic and diagnostic data from the patient population in a cardiac care unit, and assisted unit personnel in identifying a small increase in femoral access site problems following coronary angioplasty. These results led to collaborative practice review by physicians and nurses, and specific unit practice changes were then designed to impact on delivery of care.

A peer review concurrent QA audit was described by Evans and Heggie (1988), in which the intensive care units moved from an individual nurse peer review approach to a unit peer review system. This change required staff education and staff involvement and was spearheaded by clinical specialists in the critical care area.

The need to move from evaluating documentation to monitoring actual patient care is evidenced in a clinical example related to skin care, a common problem in critical care units. A survey form was developed at The University of Iowa Hospitals and Clinics for objective measurement of skin breakdown on admission and discharge from the surgical intensive care units. This tool resulted in further evaluation of patient care, a review of existing standards of skin care, and prevention of decubitus ulcers (Robnett, 1986).

Perhaps the most insightful study to link quality assurance and critical care is that of Knaus, Draper, Wagner, and Zimmerman (1986) at The George Washington University, which looked specifically at patient outcome. Intensive care units at 13 hospitals (treating approximately 5,000 patients) were studied. Knaus and the others found a significant difference in patient mortality when they used a standardized measurement tool: the Acute Physiology and Chronic Health Evaluation (APACHE) system. APACHE uses (1) acute physiology measures, (2) acute severity-of-disease measures, (3) chronic health measures, and (4) what the researchers called physiologic reserve—the ability of the individual patient to withstand an acute illness.

This particular study of quality and patient outcomes may be of paramount importance in the development of a QA model and plan for critical care units. The findings suggest that although some patients had similar APACHE scores, the predicted mortality rate was very different among the 13 hospitals studied. Upon further investigation, a questionnaire identified that the hospital variables affecting predictive mortality as measured by APACHE were a result of the individual organizational structures within the critical care units, and not the patient's status. Hospitals with a mortality rate that correlated with APACHE had the following characteristics: (1) a good system for the organization and delivery of intensive care, (2) a division of responsibility between physicians and nurses, and (3) specific protocols and standards that guided practice in a collaborative effort. Hospitals with an inverse relationship between APACHE and mortality had distrust and miscommunication between physicians and nurses. This classic study provides a conceptual framework for the development of a collaborative QA practice model that measures care within the context of standards for the critically ill.

A collaborative model for critical care units can be facilitated and supported by (1) open communication, evidenced by multidisciplinary committee membership of physicians and nurses so that standards, policies, and methods for patient care evaluation can be developed and reviewed jointly; (2) a multidisciplinary QA plan, as evidenced by clinical monitors that evaluate patient care and resultant patient outcomes from a holistic approach, rather than solely from a medical or a nursing perspective; and (3) a department management philosophy that empowers the staff nurse to be an equal partner in making decisions about patient care.

In order for these qualities and characteristics of collaborative practice to exist in critical care units or other areas in a hospital, administrative support must be evidenced by a decentralized and participative organizational structure that encourages decision making and problem resolution at the level closest to the patient. This model facilitates communication among those who are directly involved with patient care and treatment, thus making those who have the greatest potential for impact responsible and accountable for problem resolution and quality assessment. Systems that are driven by top-level decision making or that permit physicians or other departments to make independent decisions about the delivery of patient care without nursing input (or vice versa) prevent a collaborative focus in critical care.

NURSING STANDARDS IN CRITICAL CARE

The AACN published the first edition of the Standards for Nursing Care of the Critically Ill in 1981, based on Lang's QA model. The model was viewed as open and circular and provided (1) a mechanism to identify values, structure, and process; and (2) outcome standards and criteria necessary to measure the degree of attainment of standards and criteria, to interpret strengths and weaknesses based on these measurements, to identify possible courses of action, and to choose and take a final course of action (AACN, 1986). The second edition of the Standards for Nursing Care of the Critically Ill (published in 1989) builds on the previous standards, but now encompasses Donabedian's (1986) model of quality. The elements of this model include process of care delivery, outcome of care or final product, and structure or environmental components. This multidimensional approach allows for measurement of the sum of the parts since interrelationships exist among them and facilitates measurement of the three elements of critical care nursing: the critical care nurse, the critically ill patient and family, and the critical care environment.

The second edition of AACN Standards presents process and structure standards related to the critically ill. AACN has recently developed patient-centered outcome standards, which will fulfill all three elements of Donabedian's QA model: structure, process, and outcome standards (AACN, 1990). Whether standards are based on process, structure, outcome, nursing process, or body system needs, the same dilemma is present: How do we make nursing standards, regardless of their origin, valuable to nursing practice?

There is little need to duplicate work already done, but there is a need for staff to have input and ownership into the development of their unit-specific standards. Ideally, the professional staff nurse "owns" the standard and service; they are no longer the sole property or responsibility of the institution or organization (Porter-O'Grady, 1986). It is important that health care organizations move closer to standards and frameworks developed by national nursing entities such as the AACN; this move or acceptance of national standards will provide consistent methods and criteria for measuring and evaluating nursing practice.

Moreover, it is crucial that professional nurses have input into the adoption process and that individualization of these national standards occurs so that the change in ownership from institution to nurse is actualized. In enhancing the role of accountability in practice, the nurse takes on responsibility for defining the standard, adhering to the standard, and applying the standard in clinical practice, all for the benefit of patient care and outcome. Clearly, the critical care environment demands a consistent standards approach to support the very complex model of nursing care that is delivered to patients and families.

THE CRITICAL CARE QA COMMITTEE

Establishing a critical care QA committee is essential in creating a support structure that can measure and evaluate patient care in these very specialized areas. To facilitate collaboration, the committee membership should be multidisciplinary and may include staff nurses, management representation, a physician/intensivist, and other ancillary department representatives such as pharmacy, respiratory therapy, and dietary staff. This assures that key personnel who must work together as a team are sitting down together at the same table to assess the delivery and level of care given to the critically ill patient.

This participative approach helps to broaden each individual's understanding about the purpose and potential impact of QA by providing a forum for discussion and an opportunity for input. It may also persuade the caregivers to consider how the various components of patient care overlap and intersect with each other to produce quality patient outcomes. If we are to successfully assess quality and evaluate patient care, these relationships should be reflected in the multidisciplinary clinical criteria that quantify patient outcome. Thus, a multidisciplinary committee can effectively define these relationships, establish criteria that mirror these relationships, and ultimately promote a continuum of care for the patient, rather than fragments of care.

The purpose, then, of the critical care nursing QA committee is to assist in the development of these clinical monitors with measurable criteria, enabling the review and evaluation of the three components of critical care: the critical care nurse, the critically ill patient and family, and the critical care environment. In order to meet this objective, the scope of care and important aspects must be defined and understood by the committee members. The delineation process requires identifying the patient population treated in the unit(s) and selecting those critical elements of care, based on patient population, that have a potential to affect patient outcome. The following statement by Sherry Gehring, RN, Nursing Manager, reflects a potential scope of care statement that might assist the QA committee in topic development and committee direction:

The Methodist Hospital of Indiana Adult Critical Care Unit is a 22-bed, adult, medical-surgical critical care unit specializing in the care of trauma victims and liver transplant patients. The unit's population also includes burn victims and respiratory failure, overdose, renal, and cardiac patients, as well as a variety of patients requiring intense monitoring following surgical interventions. Length of stay in the unit is averaging 3.5–5.5 days, with 98 + admissions per month.

This statement, or one similar to it, should assist the QA committee in developing a specific QA plan with a purpose statement and measurable objectives based on the patient population. A yearly QA calendar for clinical monitors, with designated time periods for monitoring, can become an action plan and quick reference for the committee (see Exhibit 5-1).

The QA committee chairperson should create and establish a supportive environment that is conducive to committee members' desires to question, challenge, and explore alternatives with standards of care, practice, or policies. It is within this expansive atmosphere that clinical indicators can be developed, practice is monitored, and recommendations can be made that benefit the patient and the profession of nursing. Establishing meaningful QA monitors is a slow, evolutionary process for any QA committee. The highly technological environment and the frequent documentation requirements found in critical care can easily promote a QA process that becomes nothing more than a ''paper exercise,'' with little value to the professional nurse and others, unless a concerted effort is made to focus on human relations and behavior as they relate to the patient care delivery. In order to avoid this common pitfall, an ongoing evaluation of the clinical monitors and their ability to measure patient outcome versus tasks should be a part of the value assessment of any QA program.

For example, topics that are routinely monitored in critical care units include routine frequency data, volume indicators, adherence to nursing procedures, transfers, and adverse events. If this is the only approach to quality assurance, it can be viewed as a repetitious paper chase without value to the already too busy staff nurse. Instead, feedback is needed on more innovative topics that relate directly to the daily delivery of care. Preventing excessive blood loss in the critical care patient due to lab draws, reducing stress for the patient during the mechanical ventilation weaning process, and determining predictive factors for skin breakdown are examples of issues relevant to critical care clinical practice. The development, then, of pertinent QA monitors is a direct result of focused nursing discussions about patient care. These discussions lead to the development of clinical monitors that track and trend clinical data, identify problems, reveal areas for quality improvement, and provide an outlet for the resolution of practice concerns related to patient care.

For example, reintubation within 48 hours of extubation is an aspect of care that can be evaluated using a multidisciplinary approach. This topic was discussed at a QA retreat where staff nurses brought up the concern of the number of reintubations being performed in critical care and whether or not this was related to nursing and/or physician assessments prior to extubation. While discussing possible cause-and-effect relationships, a set of variables was generated to incorporate in a clinical monitor that measures criteria related to medical treatment, nursing assessments, and respiratory treatment. These criteria reflect a multidisciplinary look at several potential causes of or contributors to reintubation in the critically ill patient (see Exhibit 5-2).

Among the committee's primary roles are determining the appropriateness of clinical monitors and assuring that the QA data are effectively communicated back to the staff and management for timely follow-up, interventions, or changes in practice. If staff nurses are to recognize and value their participation in the process of quality assurance, management must demonstrate its willingness to act on meaningful QA data in order to "entrench" quality improvement into daily patient care. Brannon and Bucher (1989) describe quality assurance and effective nurse management as intersecting goals and observe that objective feedback derived from QA data is a potentially powerful means of enhancing nurses' performance and job satisfaction. Monitoring and measuring data are only the initial steps. The facts that nurses value feedback data and that such data can improve performance and quality, effect behavior change, and retain nurses in the system or department are well documented in the literature. A causal modeling survey of 1,597 nurses in 15 hospitals suggested that individual nurse perceptions about the quality of care

Exhibit 5-1 Critical Care Quality Assessment Yearly Calendar

CLINICAL TOPIC	JAN	FEB	MAR	APR
Admissions	X			
Sedation	X			
ET Insertion	X			
Isolation		X		
Pain Medication		X		
Pressure Set–Up		X		
Yeast Infection			X	
Oximetrix 3 Comp. HP	X		X	
Respiratory Alarms HP				X
Drawing Mixed Venous Gases				X
Transfer				
C.O. Using SAM				
Recap Needles				
AV Shunt Patency and Hemofilter				
Pleurevac/Chest Tubes				
LADD ICP				
Camino Set–Up				
Accu–chek				
Reintubation				
Intraventricular Drain Set–Up				
Blood loss via Phlebotomy				
Art Line vs. Non–Invasive Monitoring				
Completeness of Orientation	X			

Source: Courtesy of Critical Care Department, Methodist Hospital of Indiana, Inc., Indianapolis, IN.

					Year:		
MAY	JUN	JUL	AUG	SEP	OCT	NOV	DEC
		X					
		X					
	X				X	X	X
			X				
							X
							X
			X				X
X						X	
X							
	X						X
	X						
		X					
			X				
				X			
				X			
				X			
					X		
					X		
						X	
							X

Exhibit 5-2 Critical Care Clinical Monitor

Clinical Monitor: Reintubation
Indicator: Patient reintubated within
48 hours of extubation

Dx:_____   Volume: 10 patients per unit
Pt. ID # _____   Frequency: Q 6 months
Pt. Age _____

Check time frame between extubation and reintubation:
___ 12-24 hours   ___ 24-36 hours
___ 36-48 hours

Check any item that was assessed prior to extubation:
(refer to nurses notes, physician progress notes, RT
notes, lab sheet)

___ ABG   ___ Breath sounds
___ Glascow Coma Scale   ___ other: list
___ Chest x-ray   ___ Respiratory rate
___ Volumes

Vent setting prior to extubation:

FIO2 _____   Mode _____
Rate _____   Tidal Volume _____

Which group of physicians extubated patient?

___ Intensivist   ___ Pulmonologist
___ Other - list:

How many days was patient intubated? _____

What was frequency of suctioning prior to extubation?
Type of secretions and volume.

___ Q1   ___ thin   ___ small   ___ yellow ___ clear
___ Q2   ___ thick   ___ medium   ___ green   ___ labs
___ Q4   ___ frothy ___ large   ___ clear   ___ rhonchi
___ Q8   ___ white
___ Other   ___ Other

List any acute pulmonary changes prior to extubation:

___ Chest tube (List # and   ___ Pneumonia
___ Infiltrates   reason for this)   ___ Fever > 101
___ Atelectasis   ___ Other (list)

Size of tube _____
Nasal or oral _____

Did patient receive any racemic epinephrine or steroids
prior to extubation?   yes   no

Source: Courtesy of Critical Care Quality Assurance Committee, Methodist Hospital of Indiana, Inc.,
Indianapolis, IN.

being provided were significant in predicting turnover intentions (Hinshaw, Smeltzer, & Atwood, 1987).

Drawing from this information, the critical care department and the QA committee can collaboratively move the QA process from measurement concerns to staff improvement, bringing about behavior change through meaningful objective feedback.

SHAPING CLINICAL MONITORS: A CLINICAL EXAMPLE

Developing clinical monitors that measure and focus on quality improvement is a challenge. The process can be the result of formal committee meetings, brainstorming retreats, or simply an attempt to create a positive problem resolution approach to complaints voiced by staff nurses. The process can take several attempts before it is completed, it can never reach the idea stage, or it can occur so rapidly that one can barely write down the criteria quickly enough. Regardless of the development method used, the value of the clinical monitor can be evaluated on the basis of its ability to measure patient outcome according to predetermined criteria.

The criteria are developed through focused nursing discussions about patient care where individual clinical experiences, hypotheses, anecdotes, and research data may be drawn into the discussion and used to measure a "window" of patient care. One such example illustrates the creation of a clinical monitor designed to measure the "quality" or reliability of pulmonary capillary wedge pressure (PCWP) readings in the Methodist Hospital of Indiana (MHI) Critical Care department.

The critical care staff nurses had identified the problem of individual variations in PCWP readings among physicians, nurses, and preceptors in the department. This aspect of care and clinical judgment was further complicated by the ability of the cardiac monitor to calculate an automated PCWP reading from a computerized algorithm, resulting in a total of four potential interpretations. However, the MHI critical care nursing standards did not support use of the automated wedge reading in practice.

This clinical practice issue has the potential to directly affect patient outcome since the PCWP reading is used to determine fluid therapy in the critically ill patient. A wide variation in the individual interpretations could mean fluid imbalance.

In developing the PCWP clinical monitor, we recognized that certain pre-existing conditions could affect the variability of the wedge interpretation. Valvular heart disease, tachycardia, high PEEP settings on the ventilator, and cardiac dysrhythmia were known to result in high variability among readers. Therefore, rather than excluding patients with these conditions, a monitor was developed that would identify patients with these conditions, but not exclude them from the study. This attempt to include patients who were known to contribute to potential variations in interpretation allowed for identification of possible clinical conditions that might contribute to variability among readers.

Clinical information could then be used to set a nursing procedure whereby specific guidelines for interpretation of the PCWP would direct nursing practice. After the sample had been collected, the next step was to measure the variability within and among the groups. All PCWP readings were placed in a booklet so that each could be read by several individuals from the various groups. All readers were blinded from the automated monitor results.

Analysis of the data revealed minimal variability among the groups, with no relationships among experience of the reader, educational level, or shift. Most importantly, none of the patients received inappropriate fluid therapy based on the small differences among wedge readings during the concurrent tracking. The results confirmed that the "quality" of readings was much more accurate than expected and that there was little variability among the readers. Patient outcome was not affected by the individual interpretations.

Quality assurance monitors, such as in the PCWP example, measure patient outcome based on treatment or interventions. They also provide feedback to staff and management and allay the clinical concerns of staff nurses.

DESIGN OF QA FEEDBACK LOOPS

The advantage of merging quality assurance with education, objective and meaningful feedback to staff nurses, and clinical performance assessment is that the effects of specific nursing interventions can be measured by the resultant patient outcomes.

Recognizing that availability of educational resources for the professional nurse is a prerequisite to clinical performance and quality improvement, MHI's Critical Care department has established an Educational Resource Center (ERC). The ERC is located in one of the two critical care units and has more than 200 educational modules available. Topics range from nursing procedures/diagnosis, medical diagnosis or problems, and equipment to patient needs, family needs, and psychosocial determinants of care. An overlap shift time of two hours is provided so each staff nurse has ample time to complete the various modules. A given module consists of a set of instructions with a pre/post-test on the topic and explicit goals and objectives. Nurses proceed at their own pace, but completion of the module series is expected. Each successfully completed module is recorded in the staff nurse's staff development record.

The critical care clinical specialist, educator, and staff development coordinator develop the content and design the format for modules and circulate the modules to staff volunteers who review them for content validity, appropriateness, and usefulness before they are finalized and added to the series. Presentation techniques include VHS tapes, slides, cassettes, case examples with x-rays and lab results, and computer programs for self-testing. Many of the modules also contain a competency check-off component, allowing the critical care clinical specialist or educator to review the clinical performance of the nurse at the bedside. One such performance review with standardized critieria, designed to measure the nursing component of endotracheal insertion in the critical care patient, is presented in Exhibit 5-3.

The ERC is an integral part of the Critical Care department's expectations regarding clinical performance. It provides an objective, systematic way to evaluate knowledge, behavior, and clinical practice that creates an ongoing information network among the clinical practice committee, the QA program, the ERC, and the nursing standards/practice committee (see Figure 5-1). The critical care nursing standards and procedures reflect a process based on knowledge inherent in the content of the modules.

The QA committee and the management group at MHI are currently exploring ways to measure the effects of education on behavior change, clinical performance, and job satisfaction. Their investigation involves identifying variables related to individual nurse utilization of the ERC, clinical performance following module use, and effects on patient outcome.

FUTURE DIRECTIONS

The ultimate impact of quality assurance on critical care practice and patient outcome can be measured by the degree of involvement of the critical care nurse. If critical care units are to successfully create a QA plan that is valued by the staff nurse and that is of benefit to patient care, efforts must be directed toward the goal of developing a collaborative, performance-based model of nursing practice that rewards the nurse and impacts on the quality of patient outcome. Establishing a feedback loop for nurses within this performance-based model may help to improve job satisfaction and strengthen the nurse's goal-setting behavior (Locke, Shaw, Saari, & Latham, 1981). The increased goal setting can act to improve clinical performance and fulfill patient care needs.

This performance-based model implies change, and change does not just happen; it is brought about by forces within the organization or system. The current staffing shortages, low levels of job satisfaction, and rapid turnover rates in most critical care units provide additional threats to this needed change and to further advancement of an expansive QA model. However, the implementation of a QA program that is responsive to nursing and its needs may prove to be a

Exhibit 5-3 QA Monitor of Performance Criteria

Methodist Hospital OF INDIANA, INC.

ASSISTING WITH ET INSERTION

Patient ID#
Unit
Shift
Date

	Yes	No*	Comments
1. Assembles all equipment at bedside			
2. Demonstrates appropriate barrier techniques			
3. Utilizes aseptic technique			
4. Positions patient			
5. Connects O_2 flow meter			
6. Readies ambu bag			
7. Assembles suction			
8. Assesses cuff prior to insertion			
9. Assesses patient tolerance to intubation			
10. Auscultates for correct ET placement			
11. Tapes tube			
12. Obtains chest x-ray			
13. Documents procedure			

Retrospective Validation of:
Date, Time, ET Tube Size, & Location
Centimeter mark at Lip/Nares
Physician performing
Medications utilized
Vital signs
Patient tolerance
Color, amount, & consistency of suctioned
secretions
Breath sounds
O_2% and mode
Chest x-ray obtained & results
Complications & nursing interventions
Amount of tube cutoff, if any
Movement assessed and amount of air in
cuff

*Requires Comment

Source: Courtesy of Critical Care Quality Assurance Committee, Methodist Hospital of Indiana, Inc., Indianapolis, IN.

potentially powerful force in reducing or helping to alleviate some of these dilemmas currently facing most health care systems.

Hospitals are likely to try a variety of patient care models in the 1990s and beyond in order to adapt to society's ever-changing needs and attitudes (Mayer, Madden, & Lawrenz, 1990). It is clear that quality improvement will become an

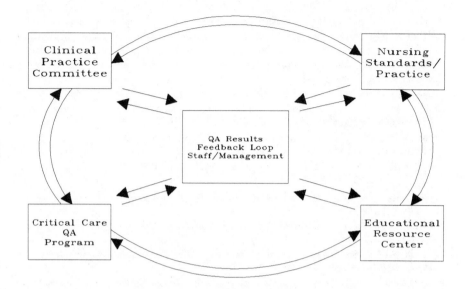

Figure 5-1 A Conceptual Model Representing the Continuous Flow of Feedback

external expectation for the various health care delivery models in light of the guidelines recently published by the Joint Commission on Accreditation of Healthcare Organizations. In addition, nurses are likely to be held professionally accountable by their peers, consumers, and the organization for evaluating the outcomes of their own practice. Nurses should be included in this change process by redefining and articulating what is best for their patients, families, and the profession of nursing. For nurses to be instrumental in the future direction of quality assurance and the advancement of a professional practice model that benefits patient care, we must each assume the responsibility for participation, development, and advancement.

REFERENCES

AACN (1990). Outcome Standards for Nursing Care of the Critically Ill. Laguna Niguel, CA: Author.

AACN. (1986). *Scope of critical care nursing practice*. Newport Beach, CA: Author.

AACN. (1981). Standards for nursing care of the critically ill. (1981). Newport Beach, CA: Author.

Bozett, F.W., & Gibbons, R. (1983). The nursing management of families in the critical care setting. *Critical Care Update*, 22–27.

Brannon, D., & Bucher, J.A. (1989). Quality assurance feedback as a nursing management strategy. *Hospitals, 34*(4), 547–558.

Carpenito, L.J. (1983). *Nursing diagnosis: Application to clinical practice*. Philadelphia: J.B. Lippincott.

Donabedian, A. (1986). Criteria and standards of quality assessment and monitoring. *Quality Review Bulletin, 12*(3), 99–108.

Evans, E., & Heggie, J. (1988). Implementing a continuous unit specific quality assurance monitor. *Journal of Quality Assurance, 2*(2), 16–23.

Gawlinski, A. (1982). Quality assurance and standards of care in the critical care setting. *Critical Care Quarterly*, 43–49.

Hinshaw, A., Smeltzer, C.H., & Atwood, J. (1987). Innovative retention strategies for nursing staff. *Journal of Nursing Administration, 17*(6), 8–16.

Knaus, W., Draper, E., Wagner, D.P., & Zimmerman, J.E. (1986). An evaluation of outcome from intensive care in major medical centers. *Annuals of Internal Medicine, 104*, 410–418.

Joint Commission on Accreditation of Healthcare Organizations. (1990). 1991 *Joint Commission Accreditation manual for hospitals* (vols I, II). Chicago: authors.

Locke, E.A., Shaw, K.N., Saari, L.M., & Latham, G.P. (1981). Goal setting and task performance. *Psychological Bulletin, 90*(1), 125–152.

Mayer, G.G., Madden, M.J., & Lawrenz, E. (1990). *Patient care delivery models.* Gaithersburg, MD: Aspen Publishers.

Pinkerton, S.E., & Schroeder, P. (1988). *Commitment to excellence: Developing a professional nursing staff.* Gaithersburg, MD: Aspen Publishers.

Porter-O'Grady, T. (1986). *Creative nursing administration: Participative management into the 21st century.* Gaithersburg, MD: Aspen Publishers.

Robnett, M.K. (1986). The incidence of skin breakdown in a surgical intensive care unit. *Journal of Nursing Quality Assurance*, 77–81.

Rowe, M.A., & Jackson, J.D. (1989). Multidisciplinary QA in critical care unit. *Journal of Nursing Quality Assurance, 3*(2), 35–40.

Sanford, S.J., & Disch, J.M. (1989). *American Association of Critical Care Nurses. Standards for nursing care of the critically ill* (2nd ed.). Norwalk, CT: Appleton & Lange.

Schroeder, P., & Maibusch, R.M. (1984). *Nursing quality assurance: A unit based approach.* Gaithersburg, MD: Aspen Publishers.

6

Monitoring Practice: A Long-Term Care Example

Tari V. Miller, RN, MS, Former Assistant Administrator/Resident Care, Lakeland Nursing Home of Walworth County, Elkhorn, Wisconsin

Marilyn J. Rantz, RN, MSN, NHA, Administrator, Lakeland Nursing Home of Walworth County, Elkhorn, Wisconsin

MONITORING AND EVALUATION FOR LONG-TERM CARE—AN EVOLVING EXAMPLE

Quality assurance (QA) activities improve patient care and fulfill the nurse's obligation of individual and collective accountability for nursing practice. The QA activities used to evaluate the effectiveness of patient care have become a requirement for both the reimbursement of services and the accreditation of health care agencies. This holds true for health care delivered in many settings, including long-term care (LTC).

It is the intent of this chapter to discuss the quality concept and quality indicators in long-term care. The primary emphasis here will be on relevant issues and strategy designs for QA monitoring specific to long-term care. Some of the concepts that will be presented include interdisciplinary quality assurance, paraprofessional staff involvement in quality assurance, and methods to disseminate and operationalize study findings.

Application of these key issues will be demonstrated through examples from the QA monitoring and evaluation system at Lakeland Nursing Home, a 328-bed, skilled, nonprofit county-operated nursing facility for long-term care. When its QA program was begun in the 1970s, the primary focus was basic compliance with regulations, mandated by state and federal legislation. With the American Nurses' Association (ANA) conceptual model as its foundation, the system has evolved into an essential mechanism for identifying and solving problems and monitoring the attainment of standards of nursing practice as defined by the professionals establishing such standards (American Nurses' Association, 1982). Quality assurance activities are now extending into broader arenas of assessment and evaluation where standards have not yet been determined in order to facilitate establishment of new practice standards.

WHAT CONSTITUTES QUALITY IN LONG-TERM CARE?

The concept of quality is an elusive, abstract concept, which health care professionals have struggled to define. The Joint Commission on Accreditation of Healthcare Organizations (1989) has defined patient care quality as "the degree to which patient/resident care services increase the probability of desired patient/ resident outcomes and reduce the probability of undesired outcomes, given the current state of knowledge" (p. 11). Because quality in long-term care must address the important issue of quality of life, the Joint Commission expands the definition of quality to include this issue. Quality of life is a multidimensional concept that includes such things as ability to participate in the activities of daily living, physical comfort, emotional well-being, and the right to self-determination.

McElroy and Herbelin (1989) view the concept of quality in long-term care as being constituted of a multitude of components. These include the client's satisfaction with the care, efficacy of care, technical proficiency and performance of care providers, accessibility and continuity of care, and cost effectiveness. As a composite, these three definitions provide a more tangible picture of the notion of quality for long-term care.

The inherent problem in determining quality standards for LTC is tied to the absence of information regarding patient dependency and the expected illness trajectory for infirmities that cannot be cured. We have developed enormous data banks of information describing acute care from which standards for expected outcomes have been derived. These data bases and subsequent care standards have not been as well defined for LTC clients who primarily exhibit chronic illnesses. Chronic illnesses have multiple possible outcomes that complicate establishing standards from which to ascertain attainment of quality. When is death the appropriate outcome, and when is it an indicator of substandard care? When is skin breakdown an inevitable outcome to be expected in a patient's chronic illness course, and when is it an indicator of inadequate care delivery? When do the patient's chronic illness and pain experience supersede maintaining full range of motion?

Let us consider the patient's right to select options for the management of his/ her course of treatment. Our experience has been that when patients are encouraged to make their own informed choices about their treatment regime, they frequently choose traditionally conservative options such as not inserting a nasogastric tube and not submitting themselves to resuscitation. However, these choices have an inevitable impact on death rate statistics. What about the patient's right to a restraint-free environment as mandated in the Omnibus Budget Reconciliation Act of 1987? Restraints have traditionally been used to attempt to provide as "safe" an environment as possible for patients who have been identified at high risk for falls. Much nursing research has been devoted to identifying those who are at high risk; however, other interventions will need to be developed and tested to avoid the use of restraints. As these are investigated and implemented, fall statistics may increase.

INDICATORS OF QUALITY IN LONG-TERM CARE

The clinical focus of quality indicators in long-term care must be conceptualized as "care" versus "cure." In the previous section, we noted that the management of nonacute chronic illness is the predominant service in long-term care. This prevalence is sharply contrasted in the acute care arena where the primary focus is cure. It is obvious that chronic illness by its very nature cannot be cured. The manifestations of these chronic disease processes are ongoing and continuous; therefore, the focus of nursing care must be on maintenance, promotion, supportive, and prevention activities when a patient experiences an inevitable illness decline. The clinical focus of care is the predominant perspective of nursing and is the appropriate framework for LTC quality assurance. Adopting the acute care focus on cure, which is the primary perspective of medicine, will interfere with the development of nursing care standards pertinent to the care being delivered in this setting.

Having eliminated cure as the usual outcome for patients receiving long-term nursing care, the quality indicators can be generated from the care framework. These indicators can be identified along a continuum ranging from specific goal attainment by individual patients to collective information about the general LTC facility, population, and industry (see Figure 6-1). For individual patients, the establishment of time-oriented, single-focused, measurable goals provides an individual standard for evaluation of the effectiveness of nursing care delivered to a given patient. Moving along the continuum, a specific nursing intervention being delivered to a group of patients with a similar response to a health care problem can be evaluated for overall effectiveness. At the latter end of the spectrum, aggregate

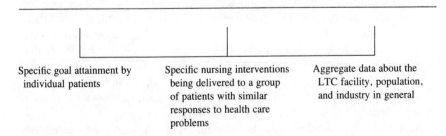

| Specific goal attainment by individual patients | Specific nursing interventions being delivered to a group of patients with similar responses to health care problems | Aggregate data about the LTC facility, population, and industry in general |

Figure 6-1 Continuum of Quality Indicators. *Source:* Courtesy of Lakeland Nursing Home, Elkhorn, WI.

data may be analyzed to identify potential standards by which care delivery could be measured.

RELEVANT ISSUES AND STRATEGY DESIGNS SPECIFIC TO LONG-TERM CARE

To actuate changes in nursing practice based on QA study findings, action strategies must be formalized and innovations stabilized within the organization. The remainder of this chapter will focus on relevant issues and strategy designs for QA monitoring with specific emphasis to long-term care.

Regulatory Agency Impact versus a Professional Practice QA Model

In the LTC industry, QA monitoring is governed by mandates in state codes and related federal legislation. The Omnibus Reconciliation Act of 1987 (1989) further expands on current mandates and requires skilled nursing facilities to "maintain a quality assessment and assurance committee consisting of the director of nursing services; a physician designated by the facility; and at least three other members of the facility's staff. The quality assurance and assessment committee meets at least quarterly to identify issues with respect to which quality assessment and assurance activities are necessary; and develops and implements appropriate plans of action to correct identified quality deficiencies." The focus of a QA monitoring program based on these legal parameters is on compliance with regulations, as opposed to a QA monitoring program based on a professional practice model and eventual patient care outcomes. One system being tested by regulators and LTC facilities in New York is based on QA outcome measures as well as regulations (Shaw & Whelan, 1989). The system evaluates 12 clinical outcome areas designed to focus on patient risk factors as well as required surveillance issues.

It is interesting to note that the impact of regulatory agencies on the development of QA assessment and monitoring in long-term care subsequent to the OBRA 1987 legislation somewhat parallels the development of QA monitoring in acute care subsequent to Joint Commission requirements. As a QA program evolves from a professional practice model, professionals identify problem issues related to the care they are delivering, take corrective action, and continually monitor for the effectiveness of alternative strategies. This approach facilitates the constant development, revision, and evolution of the practice discipline.

Now that quality assessment has been mandated in long-term care, one has to be concerned whether the findings of a QA committee can be used by regulatory agencies in a punitive way. If that is indeed the case, the focus of the QA issues and problems the committee may identify and address will change. It is imperative to bear in mind that the ultimate purpose of a QA monitoring program is to assure the consumer or client that we as a nursing profession are continually evaluating and improving our knowledge and skills in order to provide excellent nursing care. Historically, the intent of QA audits has been exactly that: to improve the quality of care and reassure consumers either directly or indirectly. If regulatory agencies focus on the punitive, the evolution of the professional practice model will stop, and staff acceptance and recognition of QA study findings are going to be minimized—and may, in fact, have a negative connotation.

An example of this regulatory versus practice dilemma that we have encountered in our own agency is related to patients identified as being highly prone to fall. In our agency, a "potential for physical injury" care plan is initiated when a patient is identified at high risk for falls. This plan is highly specific and delineates individualized interventions to reduce each patient's risk for falls and maintain independence. During our last state survey process, a specific patient who was identified at high risk for falls attracted particular attention and in-depth investigation because the data that we had been monitoring were readily available and being actively dealt with by the nursing staff. The staff perceived this investigation as negative. This becomes an obvious dilemma for practitioners. When a patient care problem is identified and monitored through QA activities, we need the professional freedom to deal with the issue and not be restrained by the fear of reprisal.

Interdisciplinary Quality Assurance

Interdisciplinary quality assurance has several potential benefits, including a focus on overall patient care by all ancillary disciplines involved in delivery of that care, facilitation of multidisciplinary communication, and recognition of each individual discipline's contribution to a patient's total care. Interdisciplinary QA studies may be interdepartmental in nature, or they may be simply a nursing department study with input and/or asssistance from ancillary disciplines. Other disciplines may also perform studies focusing on a singular aspect of care delivered by each specific discipline. In our agency, the therapeutic recreation department conducts approximately four QA studies annually. It evaluates such things as the types of therapeutic recreation programs being delivered to patients, the appropriateness of these activities based on individual, patient-identified leisure interests, and studies that objectively validate they are offering the minimum number of programs per patient per week as mandated by the state code.

An example of a multidisciplinary QA study that is conducted biannually is the patient admission/readmission assessment audit. This audit is designed to ascertain compliance with mandated admission/readmission assessment data within specified time frames. All disciplines involved in direct patient care (nursing, social services, therapeutic recreation, dietary, occupational therapy, physical therapy, and speech therapy as prescribed) are mandated in the state of Wisconsin to perform an admission/readmission assessment within 72 hours for nursing, and within two weeks for all other disciplines, following a patient's admission to the facility. This QA study has been designed from a multidisciplinary perspective with a simple auditing tool to review the charts of all patients admitted during the study period of evaluation to assure the appropriate assessments have been completed on a timely basis with corresponding signatures, dates, etc. (see Exhibit 6-1).

An ongoing QA monitoring methodology within our agency is the inter-disciplinary care planning process. On a quarterly basis, the care plan of each patient in our facility is reviewed by all disciplines involved in care delivery. At that time, all identified problems for each individual patient are reviewed, and the established long-term and short-term interdisciplinary goals are reviewed for appropriateness and attainment. This area is frequently overlooked as a QA monitoring activity, but we view it as an essential component of the overall QA umbrella.

Centralized versus Decentralized Quality Assurance

The ultimate purpose of QA activities is to constantly improve the care activities that have been the focus of the QA study. In order to legitimize QA study findings and establish accountability for subsequent follow-through with these findings, formal organizational linkages must be established (Miller & Rantz, 1989). In practice, many facilities simply identify a QA coordinator in a staff role with no line accountability or responsibility for direct nursing care. Stevens (1983) notes that direct lines of authority establish formal chains of command and create a legitimate span of control that can facilitate change implementation.

A major deterrent to using a staff person as a QA coordinator is the potential for that person to become the sole responsible party for all QA activities. It is important that members throughout the organization participate in the QA process. Such involvement is facilitated by the use of a participative committee structure, rather than locating all QA activities centrally with one figure. The participative principle facilitates the entire QA monitoring process by virtue of the fact that the people doing the monitoring are also those delivering the care and they are actually monitoring compliance with their own practice, as opposed to having an outside individual tell them about their practice.

The organizational structure we have implemented to stabilize actual practice changes is designed to provide a formal link among our QA Committee, Policy and Procedure Committee, and nursing administration. In our LTC setting, the nursing administrator chairs both the Policy and Procedure Committee and the QA

Exhibit 6-1 Patient Admission/Readmission Assessment Audit

DISCIPLINE _____ Nursing

RESIDENT	ADMISSION DATE	AREA	Within 72 hours of resident's admission to Lakeland Nursing Home, a nursing manager/ coordinator or designee has supervised the preparation of a written history and assessment summarizing the resident's prior health and disabilities (Nursing Health Patterns Assessment Tool).			The signature of the person completing the admission assessment is on the assessment form in the designated area. (A registered nurse must cosign admission assessment forms completed by LPNs).		The date of the admission assessment is on the assessment form in the designated area.		CORRECTIVE ACTION TAKEN AS INDICATED			COMMENTS
			YES	NO	N/A	YES	NO	YES	NO	YES	NO	N/A	

DISCIPLINE Social Services, Therapeutic Recreation, Dietary, Physical Therapy, Occupational Therapy, Speech Therapy

continues

Exhibit 6-1 continued

RESIDENT	ADMISSION DATE	AREA	Within 2 weeks of resident's admission to Lakeland Nursing Home, all disciplines involved in delivery of care to the resident have prepared a written history and assessment.			The signature of the person completing the admission assessment is on the assessment form in the designated area.		The date of the admission assessment is on the assessment form in the designated area.		CORRECTIVE ACTION TAKEN AS INDICATED			COMMENTS
			YES	NO	N/A	YES	NO	YES	NO	YES	NO	N/A	

Source: Courtesy of Lakeland Nursing Home, Elkhorn, WI.

Committee. This arrangement provides a direct sanction from nursing administration for all policy and procedure decisions based on QA study findings that affect direct patient care. The nursing management staff reporting to the nursing administrator is responsible for ensuring compliance with these subsequent practice changes. While the formal linkage is centralized with the nursing administrator, the committee activities are conducted by highly involved nurse participants.

Paraprofessional Staff Involvement in Quality Assurance

Nursing practice changes that result from QA studies must be disseminated to all personnel levels in the department of nursing. In the LTC setting, this is significant to nurse assistants because they are, in fact, providing direct patient care and comprise the majority of actual nursing staff. Quality assurance study findings and related policy and procedure revisions in our agency are disseminated to this group in monthly nurse assistant staff meetings conducted by nursing administration on all three shifts. Additionally, a monthly Nurse Assistant Practice Committee meeting addresses patient practice concerns. This committee, as well as nurse assistant volunteers, may actually be involved in QA data retrieval and may contribute subsequent recommendations for follow-up action. Again, involvement of this level of nursing staff in actual QA auditing encourages staff support and increases their recognition of the need for practice changes.

A relevant example of paraprofessional involvement in an ongoing QA study in our agency is reflected in our concurrent audit tool for charting. Exhibit 6-2 is page 1 of our nurse assistant documentation tool, and the corresponding audit tool is found in Exhibit 6-3. This audit tool has been designed to objectively measure compliance with documentation of nurse assistance care delivery to patients on a daily basis as delineated on their LTC flow sheet. The study is conducted on a monthly basis by an assigned nurse assistant on each shift. The findings are then reviewed by the area unit nurse and presented at a monthly unit conference with all nurse assistants assigned to that unit.

Another relevant example of paraprofessional involvement in QA monitoring can be seen in a recent QA study that evaluated nursing staff's awareness of and compliance with patient grooming and hygiene needs. The overall study objectives were to (1) identify relevant areas of strength or deficiency in meeting patient grooming and hygiene needs and (2) propose feasible alternatives for corrective intervention or progress changes in order to improve the quality of care in these areas. Again, representatives from the Nurse Assistant Practice committee assisted the QA Committee in retrieving data for this study. The data consisted of observations on specific elements of patient grooming and hygiene. Audit criteria included a subjective evaluation of such items as the patient's general appearance, hair grooming, fingernail condition, and proper fit of personal attire. Following

Exhibit 6-2 Long-Term Care Record

MONTH/YEAR _____

NUTRITIONAL-METABOLIC
PATTERN

KEY: Ab = Absent from facility, except for hospitalization; H = Hospital—mark initial day of leave to hospital. Draw line through the days of hospital stay.

BASIC NUTRITION	BREAKFAST	1	2	3	4	5	6	7	8	9	10	11	12	13	14	15	16	17	18	19	20	21	22	23	24	25	26	27	28	29	30	31
"HOW" KEY: R = Refused;	HOW																															
N = NPO; Sy = Syringe;	WHERE																															
P = Partial Assist; T = Total	AMOUNT																															
Assist	LUNCH																															
Self (may leave	HOW																															
"HOW" calendar blank)	WHERE																															
Feeding Tube	AMOUNT																															
"WHERE" KEY: U = Unit;	SUPPER																															
D = Dining Room; RT = RT	HOW																															
Activity; H = Hospital	WHERE																															
Amt/Food Intake: 0-100%	AMOUNT																															

NUTRITIONAL SUPPLEMENT

SUPPLEMENTS		1	2	3	4	5	6	7	8	9	10	11	12	13	14	15	16	17	18	19	20	21	22	23	24	25	26	27	28	29	30	31
KEY: 0-100% = Supplement	DAYS																															
Taken; R = Refused;	PMs																															
OU = OffUnit	NOCs																															
Nutritional																																	

Supplement Liquid
_____ Amt. _____ Freq.

NUTRITIONAL SNACK

		1	2	3	4	5	6	7	8	9	10	11	12	13	14	15	16	17	18	19	20	21	22	23	24	25	26	27	28	29	30	31
Bedtime Snack	DAYS																															
Nutritional	PMs																															
Supplement Pudding	NOCs																															
_____ Freq.	HS SNACK																															

		1	2	3	4	5	6	7	8	9	10	11	12	13	14	15	16	17	18	19	20	21	22	23	24	25	26	27	28	29	30	31
SPECIAL SKIN CARE	DAYS																															
	PMs																															
	NOCs																															

KEY: "√" = Care Delivered;
R = Refused; NN = Nursing
Notes

Apply _____
_____ Freq _____ Site

		1	2	3	4	5	6	7	8	9	10	11	12	13	14	15	16	17	18	19	20	21	22	23	24	25	26	27	28	29	30	31
	DAYS																															
	PMs																															
	NOCs																															

Apply _____
_____ Freq _____ Site

		1	2	3	4	5	6	7	8	9	10	11	12	13	14	15	16	17	18	19	20	21	22	23	24	25	26	27	28	29	30
PERI-CARE SCHEDULED/	DAYS																														
UNSCHEDULED	PMs																														
	NOCs																														

KEY: # = Times Delivered;
R = Refused; "√" = NA
Follow-Up as Applicable;
NN = Nursing Notes
Self-Care (leave
calendar blank)

Source: Courtesy of Lakeland Nursing Home, Elkhorn, WI.

Exhibit 6-3 Concurrent Audit Tool for Charting

Criteria	Yes	No	N/A	Comments
1. *Basic Nutrition* (*Hospitalization: Put "H" on calendar on date of hospitalization. When resident returns, draw a line from "H" to current date.) a. Self box or feeding tube box is checked if applicable.				
b. "How" section of calendar is blank if self box or feeding box is checked.				
c. "How" section of calendar is completed on all other records with R = Refused, N = NPO, Sy = Syringe, P = Partial Assist, or T = Total Assist.				
d. "Where" section of calendar notes U = Unit, D = Dining room, and RT = RT activity.				
e. "Amount" section of calendar completed on all resident's eating on unit with 0–100% of food intake.				
2. *Supplements* a. Not applicable for this resident.				
b. Nutritional supplement liquid box, bedtime snack box, and/or nutritional supplement pudding box are checked if a supplement is ordered.				
c. The amount and frequency of the supplement are noted if a supplement is ordered. (Amount not indicated for nutritional pudding.)				
d. Percent of supplement taken, R = Refused, or OU = Off Unit is recorded in calendar section if supplement is ordered.				
3. *Special Skin Care* a. Not applicable for this resident.				
b. Appropriate box checked if a specific ointment/cream is ordered.				
c. The name, frequency, and site of the specific ointment/cream are recorded if ordered.				
d. The calendar section is completed related to cream application if ordered with √ = Care Delivered, R = Refused, or NN = Nursing Notes.				
e. If "NN" is recorded on a calendar, an explanatory nursing note appears in the narrative nursing notes section.				

Exhibit 6-3 continued

Criteria	Yes	No	N/A	Comments
4. *Peri-Care Scheduled/Unscheduled* a. Calendar section is completed with a record of the actual number of times peri-care was done on each shift, "√" indicates that follow-up was done on resident when indicated, R = Refused, or NN = Nursing Notes.				
b. If resident is self-care, a "√" is placed in the appropriate box in left column, and the calendar is left blank.				
c. If "NN" is recorded on calendar, the number of times peri-care delivered is also recorded (i.e., 3/NN).				
d. If "NN" is recorded on calendar, an explanatory nursing note appears in the narrative nursing notes section.				

Source: Courtesy of Lakeland Nursing Home, Elkhorn, WI.

data retrieval, both the QA Committee and the Nurse Assistant Practice Committee reviewed the results, interpreted the findings, and recommended follow-up action.

Paraprofessional staff involvement in the actual data retrieval for these types of studies has been invaluable and has added significant validity to the study findings. It is far easier to achieve compliance with such things as nurse assistant documentation or grooming and hygiene objectives when the staff delivering the care has been involved in the QA activities.

Dissemination of Audit Findings and Operationalization of Study Recommendations

Once the QA committee has recommended a course of action, an organizational structure must be in place to ensure optimal integration of QA audit findings into actual clinical nursing practice. As already discussed, the most common structure is a participative committee. Such a committee must have not only the responsibility for implementing practice changes, but also the legitimate authority to ensure that the changes take place.

In our agency, the recommendations from the QA Committee are forwarded to the appropriate committee or other organizational system for follow-up action as indicated by the study. If a major area of concern is identified, the QA Committee may recommend establishing an ad hoc steering committee to thoroughly investigate and design an appropriate action strategy. If the study findings warrant a revision in a current policy or procedure, the QA Committee makes a definitive recommendation about the actual change needed and forwards that change recommendation to the Policy and Procedure Committee for consideration and final approval. The latter committee has legitimate authority to revise and approve the recommended changes. Subsequently, it is responsible for informing all staff, usually through a written procedural format sent to each nurse in conjunction with a notification memo outlining the actual changes. To further facilitate communication, routine unit conferences that discuss procedural or policy revisions are conducted each week on the nursing units. These help disseminate related information to all levels of staff within the organization. Special inservices on major procedural or policy changes are conducted as needed for all nursing staff. Correlating with this participative committee design is the notion of a formalized linkage between these committees, as already mentioned in this chapter.

Other organizational systems used for disseminating QA findings include monthly unit nurse meetings, conducted on all three shifts by the responsible nurse managers, where information can be presented and discussed. A quarterly meeting of all licensed staff nurses has provided a forum in which nursing administration can address specific QA findings and relevant practice-related nursing issues. When all of the licensed staff nurses attend, open discussions may be generated that result in the development of an ad hoc committee to further investigate a practice area of concern.

Quality assurance findings are also discussed at biweekly nurse administrative staff meetings. These are forums in which the nurse administration meets with all of the nursing managers in the agency to address pertinent nursing practice and management issues. Quality assurance information is often disseminated from the nursing administrative staff meetings to the unit nurses via the unit nurse meetings or to the entire nursing staff via the unit conference structures already discussed.

One common method of sharing QA study findings with all staff is the unit conference tool. For an actual example of such a tool, we will refer to the patient grooming and hygiene audit previously mentioned. Upon reviewing the study results for this audit, the QA and Nurse Assistant Practice committees recommended conducting unit conferences on all three shifts for the purpose of sharing the audit findings with all nursing staff. A unit conference tool was developed to provide a formal feedback loop for the communication of audit results to the staff delivering the services. The tool displayed the composite results of the audit findings as compared to findings from a similar audit conducted during the previous year (see Table 6-1).

A memo of explanation was circulated to all unit nurses to provide direction for conducting the unit conferences, and this memo accompanied the actual unit conference tool. The memo suggested commending all nursing staff for the

Table 6-1 Quality Assurance Unit Conference Tool—Resident Grooming/Hygiene Audit

CRITERIA	TOTAL NUMBER OF OBSERVATIONS	ACTUAL NUMBER OF OBSERVATIONS OF COMPLIANCE	PERCENTAGE OF COMPLIANCE IN 8/89	FORMER PERCENTAGE OF COMPLIANCE IN 8/88
1. In general, resident appears neat, clean, and well-kempt.	130	110 (N/A = 9)	92	93
2. Resident's hair is neatly combed and groomed.	130	107 (N/A = 9)	89	83
3. Resident's face is clean and free from food particles.	130	114 (N/A = 9)	95	94
4. Male resident is clean shaven.	130	54 (N/A = 65)	92	86
5. Resident's eyeglasses are clean and properly in place, when applicable.	130	62 (N/A = 57)	92	84
6. Resident's hearing aid is properly inserted, when applicable.	130	31 (N/A = 99)	100	95
7. Resident has dentures in, when applicable.	130	75 (N/A = 52)	98	99
8. Resident's breath is fresh and free from odor.	130	111 (N/A = 6)	90	86
9. Resident's fingernails are trimmed and clean.	130	97 (N/A = 4)	78	84
10. *In general, resident's clothing fits properly.	130	124 (N/A = 1)	96	97
11. *In general, resident's clothing is clean.	130	121	93	95
12. In general, resident's clothing is in good repair (no holes, no missing buttons, functional zippers).	130	126	97	96
13. *Resident's clothing is properly buttoned, fastened, and/or zippered.	130	123	95	95

continues

Table 6-1 continued

CRITERIA	TOTAL NUMBER OF OBSERVATIONS	ACTUAL NUMBER OF OBSERVATIONS OF COMPLIANCE	PERCENTAGE OF COMPLIANCE IN 8/89	FORMER PERCENTAGE OF COMPLIANCE IN 8/88
14. Resident's clothing is properly applied (i.e., clothing is not applied "backwards").	130	125 (N/A=5)	100	99
15. Split-back gowns/clothing/pants are properly positioned on resident to avoid exposure of bare skin.	130	61 (N/A=59)	92	90
16. Undergarments not visible under resident's clothing.	130	116 (N/A=3)	92	92
17. Hospital gowns not placed under resident's clothing.	130	101 (N/A=16)	90	97
18. Female resident's stockings are pulled up properly with no visible holes.	130	77 (N/A=49)	97	92
19. Lap robe is positioned properly around the resident, when applicable.	130	42 (N/A=78)	92	97
20. Restraint is positioned properly, when applicable.	130	84 (N/A=45)	99	99
21. Resident's catheter bag is properly covered for privacy, when applicable.	130	31 (N/A=97)	99	95
22. *Foley tubing is properly draped, when applicable.	130	32 (N/A=94)	97	—
23. Resident wearing properly fastened shoes, slippers, or other appropriate attire on feet.	130	118 (N/A=8)	97	97
24. *Staff demonstrates proper hand washing between residents when delivering direct care.	130	68 (N/A=44)	86	—

*Area of concern during 1989 State Survey

Source: Courtesy of Lakeland Nursing Home, Elkhorn, WI.

obvious personalized attention they had given to meeting the patients' grooming and hygiene needs. The purposes of the unit conference were (1) to provide positive reinforcement for the excellent care being provided to the patients and (2) to increase awareness of the need to continue fulfilling patient grooming and hygiene needs in order to facilitate actual changes in care practice delivery.

As a committee, we are continually evaluating our methods for disseminating QA study findings and seeking creative ideas for sharing these results. One of our more innovative methodologies was a videotape of staff and patient vignettes, which was produced and managed by representatives from the QA and Nurse Assistant Practice committees. Although a great deal of humor was used to share the message of the audit findings, the actual study results were apparent to viewers. This was a nice diversion from some of the more routine and expected methods for sharing QA study findings, and yet it proved to be very effective and was shown to all disciplines within the facility.

Administrative Monitors of Quality

The scope of QA monitoring can encompass a wide spectrum of information. Long-term care nursing facilities already collect a wide variety of clinical and administrative data that definitely fall within the spectrum of QA monitoring. These data are frequently overlooked for this purpose and at times are collected and never analyzed. We contend that this information should be further examined and the findings evaluated as valuable indicators of quality.

Clinical data that are frequently collected in most LTC agencies include medication errors, communicable infections, incident/accident occurrences, drug utilization, and mortality. In our agency, we also maintain the frequencies of nursing diagnoses identified in our geriatric population. This allows us to observe trends that reflect changes in our population, contributes data needed for developing and validating diagnoses, and provides nurse administration with objective data for strategic management and planning (Rantz & Miller, 1987).

Most facilities collect some types of clinical statistics from a simple frequency perspective. Quality assurance studies could be designed to further evaluate these statistics and identify related areas of concern that may result from more in-depth examination. For example, during a unit reorganization, we identified a concern related to patient relocation. We re-examined the death rate data that had already been compiled from a different perspective. This analysis showed us that, in fact, relocation from one room to another room or from one area to another area did have a significant impact on accelerating the death of some patients (Rantz & Egan, 1987).

In another situation, clinical statistical information was re-examined subsequent to a patient incident/accident documentation audit that indicated an excessive number of patient falls. Based on this problem identification, an ad hoc steering committee was formulated to further investigate this paramount area of concern. The committee began by conducting a more detailed investigation of the factors surrounding the reported patient falls, whether the falls were observed or unobserved, and other related factors (i.e., use of psychotropic medications, patient condition during the shift prior to the fall, contributing environmental factors, etc.). This ad hoc committee has continued to investigate the problem and is currently examining a multitude of variables related to the problem of patients who are highly prone to fall. Again, it is significant to note that this was stimulated by a simple analysis of information that is being collected on an ongoing basis.

Other types of general administrative data collected that could be appropriately classified as quality monitors include data collected to comply with state and federal regulations. Most facilities maintain records regarding physicians' visits, admission, discharge, hospitalization, and medical diagnoses, to name a few. While we are collecting the information that enables regulatory agencies to monitor our compliance with their regulations, we can examine these data in more detail from the QA perspective, which goes beyond simple frequency monitoring.

Nurses and nurse assistants are the primary caregivers in long-term care. The Institute of Medicine report entitled *Improving the Quality of Care in Nursing Homes* (1986) revealed that one of the major factors affecting the quality of care and the quality of life in nursing homes is the number and the quality of nursing staff. All nursing homes maintain statistics concerning the hours of direct care (and indirect care) provided to their patients. These are computed in a relatively standardized fashion and reported to various state and federal agencies. The basic hours per patient per day of service statistic can function as a quality-monitoring indicator. It is a readily available statistic and can be used to compare one agency with another. Enough staff time must be provided to be able to deliver the care that the patients need. Other administrative types of data usually collected in most agencies include information concerning employee work-related injuries. Upon further examination, this information may provide structural and environmental data to the facility administration for general decision making and improvement of the safety of the agency's working conditions.

Some basic staff-related data that are traditionally collected are employee absenteeism, employee turnover, and related longevity. Conducting exit interviews following employee resignations can provide further insightful information for the facility administration to use in making decisions to improve employee retention and recruitment. The key point that we want to emphasize is that all kinds of data collected within an organization should be considered when evaluating and monitoring attainment of quality. As previously mentioned, this is often not given the time and consideration that it deserves, and yet we have found it to be invaluable in the effective management of our skilled long-term nursing facility.

CONCLUSION

Quality assurance programs in long-term care *do* provide a mechanism for continuously evaluating and improving nursing practice skills that ultimately make a clinical difference at the bedside. Inherent in an applicable long-term care QA design is the need for attention to the overall concept of quality, conceptualizing quality indicators in terms of "care," rather than "cure." It is also imperative to consider that these quality indicators are identified along a continuum ranging from individual goal attainment to collective information about the LTC facility, population, and industry in general. A QA monitoring and evaluation program must be an active, continuous, and comprehensive examination of care delivery and facility services in order to objectively ascertain the provision of high-quality care. It is essential to systematically develop a practical QA framework and supportive organizational management structures in order to optimally integrate study findings into clinical nursing and interdisciplinary practice of LTC agencies.

REFERENCES

American Nurses' Association. (1982). *Nursing quality assurance management/learning system: Professional nurses' role in quality assurance.* Kansas City, MO/Northridge, CA: Author/Sutherland.

Institute of Medicine. (1986). *Improving the quality of care in nursing homes.* Washington, DC: National Academy Press.

Joint Commission on Accreditation of Healthcare Organizations. (1989). *Quality assurance in long term care.* Chicago: Author.

McElroy, D., & Herbelin, K. (1989). Assuring quality of care in long term facilities. *Journal of Gerontological Nursing, 15*(7), 8–10.

Miller, T.V., & Rantz, M.J. (1989). Management structures to facilitate practice changes subsequent to QA activities. *Journal of Nursing Quality Assurance, 3*(4), 21–27.

Omnibus Budget Reconciliation Act of 1987. (1989, February 2). *Federal Register, 54*(21), 5,358–5,373.

Rantz, M., & Egan, K. (1987). Reducing death from translocation syndrome. *American Journal of Nursing, 87*(10), 1351–1352.

Rantz, M., & Miller, T.V. (1987). How diagnoses are changing in long-term care. *American Journal of Nursing, 87*(3), 360–361.

Shaw, J.D., & Whelan, R.E. (1989). QA outcome measures in long-term care. *Journal of Nursing Quality Assurance, 4*(1), 48–61.

Stevens, B.J. (1983). *First-line patient care management.* Gaithersburg, MD: Aspen Publishers.

SUPPLEMENTAL BIBLIOGRAPHY

American Nurses' Association. (1982). *Nursing quality assurance management/learning system: Guide for nursing quality assurance coordinators and administrators.* Kansas City, MO/Northridge, CA: Author/Sutherland.

American Nurses' Association. (1982). *Nursing quality assurance management/learning system: Workbook for nursing quality assurance committee members—long-term care facilities.* Kansas City, MO/Northridge, CA: Author/Sutherland.

Burmeister, R. (1986). Commentary: Blast or boost? *Quality Review Bulletin, 12*(12), 417–419.

Chambers, L.W., and Blum, H.M. (1988). Measurement of actions of care-providers in long-term care. *Journal of Clinical Epidemiology, 41*(8), 793–802.

Cleary, P.D., and McNeil, B.J. (1988). Patient satisfaction as an indicator of quality care. *Inquiry, 25*(1), 25–36.

Davies, A.R., and Ware, J.E. (1988). Involving consumers in quality of care assessment. *Health Affairs, 7*(1), 33–48.

Davis, B.A., and Lee, P.L. (1987). Standards of gerontological/long term care nursing practice. *Quality Review Bulletin, 13*(11), 377–379.

Donabedian, A. (1976). Some basic issues in evaluating the quality of health care. In *Issues in Evaluation Research* (pp. 3–28) (ANA Publication No. G-124). Kansas City, MO: American Nurses' Association.

Donabedian, A. (1981). Advantages and limitations of explicit criteria for assessing the quality of health care. *Quarterly/Health and Society, 59*, 99–104.

Grimaldi, P.L., Micheletti, J.A., & Shala, T.J. (1987). Quality assurance in a PaCS and case-mix environment. *Quality Review Bulletin, 13*(5), 170–174.

Grzeczkowski, A.M., & Knapp, M. (1988). The gerontological nurse practitioner as director of nursing in the long-term facility. *Nursing Management, 19*(4), 64B–64F.

Haff, J., McGowan, C., Potts, C., & Streekstra, C. (1988). Evaluating primary nursing in long-term care: Provider and consumer opinions. *Journal of Nursing Quality Assurance, 2*(3), 44–53.

Harrington, C. (1987). Nursing Home reform: Addressing critical staffing issues. *News Outlook, 35*(5), 208–209.

Hart, M.A., & Sliefert, M.K. (1983). Monitoring patient incidents in a long term care facility. *Quality Review Bulletin, 9*(12), 356–365.

Heater, B.S., Becker, A.M., & Olsen, R.K. (1988). Nursing interventions and patient outcomes; A meta-analysis of studies. *Nursing Research, 37*(5), 303–307.

Hewitt, S.M., LeSage, J., Roberts, K.L., & Ellor, J.R. (1985). Process auditing in long term care facilities. *Quality Review Bulletin, 11*(1), 6–15.

Howe, M.J. (1980). Developing instruments for measurement of criteria: A clinical nursing practice perspective. *Nursing Research, 29*(2), 100–103.

Joint Commission on Accreditation of Hospitals. (1988). *Quality assurance in long term care.* Chicago: Author.

Kane, R.A., & Kane, R.L. (1988). Long-term care: Variations on a quality assurance theme. *Inquiry, 25*(1), 132–146.

Kayser-Jones, J. (1989). The environment and quality of life in long-term care institutions. *Nursing and Health Care, 10*(3), 125–130.

Kraft, M.R., Neubauer, J.A., & LeSage, J. (1987). Quality monitoring in long-term care. *Journal of Nursing Quality Assurance, 2*(1), 39–48.

Lang, N. (1989). Non-hospital, non-physician review. *AMPRA Review, 5*(4), 1–2.

Lohr, K.N. (1988). Outcome measurement: Concepts and questions. *Inquiry, 25*(1), 37–50.

Lohr, K.N., Yordy, K.D., & Thier, S.O. (1988). Current issues in quality of care. *Health Affairs, 7*(1), 5–18.

Micheletti, J.A., & Shala, T.J. (1986). RUGs II: Implications for management and quality in long term care. *Quality Review Bulletin, 12*(7), 236–242.

Mitty, E.L. (1988). Resource utilization groups, DRGs move to long-term care. *Nursing Clinics of North America, 23*(3), 539–557.

Mohide, E.A., Caulfield, P.A., Dunnett, C.W., & Bayne, J.R. (1988). Randomized trial of quality assurance in nursing homes. *Medical Care, 26*(6), 554–565.

Pelletier, L.R., & Poster, E.C. (1988). Part 1: An overview of evaluation methodology for nursing quality assurance programs. *Journal of Nursing Quality Assurance, 2*(4), 55–62.

Peters, D.A. (1989). An overview of current research relating to long-term outcomes. *Nursing and Health Care, 10*(3), 133–136.

Poster, E.C., & Pelletier, L.R. (1988). Part 2: Quantitative and qualitative approaches to nursing quality assurance program evaluation. *Journal of Nursing Quality Assurance, 2*(4), 63–72.

Roberts, K.L., LeSage, J., & Ellor, J.R. (1987). Quality monitoring in nursing homes. *Journal of Gerontological Nursing, 13*(10), 34–40.

Roper, W.L., & Hackbarth, G.M. (1988). HCFA's agenda for promoting high-quality care. *Health Affairs, 7*(1), 91–98.

Sherrad, H. (1985). QA issues in long-term care—Vehicle for introducing change. *Dimensions in Health Services, 62*(10), 8–10.

Smeltzer, C.H. (1983). Organizing the search for excellence. *Nursing Management, 14*(6), 19–21.

Smith, D. (1988). Collaboration in nursing research—A multi-disciplinary approach. *International Journal of Nursing Studies, 25*(1), 73–78.

Stiffer federal regulation of nursing homes proposed by Institute of Medicine. (1986). *Geriatric Nursing, 7*(3), 122–124.

Vladeck, B.C., & Kramer, P.S. (1988). Case mix measures: DRGs and alternatives. *Annual Reviews Inc., 19*, 333–359.

Whiteneck, M.R. (1988). Integrating ethics with quality assurance in long term care. *Quality Review Bulletin, 14*(5), 138–143.

7

Monitoring Practice: An Ambulatory Care Example

Jane A. Miller, RN, MSN, CPQA, Quality Assurance Project Specialist, Ambulatory Care Services Department, Methodist Hospital of Indiana, Inc., Indianapolis, Indiana

The prominence of ambulatory settings in health care delivery is increasing rapidly. The "new wave" and "diversification" are the terms used by the American Hospital Association (AHA) to describe the current phase in the evolution of ambulatory care. Outpatient surgery and satellite facilities are key examples of growth that AHA cites. The AHA's hospital-sponsored ambulatory care utilization trend statistics for the five years from 1983 to 1988 (Table 7-1) provide dramatic evidence of ambulatory care growth. These figures document a phenomenon we all no doubt sense or confront directly, in both our professional and our personal interactions with the U.S. health care system.

The increasing prominence of the ambulatory setting relates not only to numbers, but also to the complexity of services. Invasive diagnostic and treatment procedures calling for sophisticated skills previously delivered only in hospital critical care units and laboratory departments are now being provided in outpatient centers and homes. Much of the education for self-care previously delivered during hospital stays now must be provided in ambulatory and home settings. Also, as increasingly sophisticated concepts of self-care are to be learned by patients and family members (people from multiple socioeconomic backgrounds with varying resources), the providers of self-care education in ambulatory settings face increasing expectations and challenges.

The term *ambulatory care* will be used to refer to health care provided to a patient in a setting other than an inpatient hospital area or the patient's home. The Joint Commission on Accreditation of Healthcare Organizations (1990) lists the following examples of ambulatory settings:

- ambulatory care clinics
- ambulatory surgery centers
- college or university health programs
- community health centers

Table 7-1 Hospital-Sponsored Ambulatory Care Utilization Trends (1983–1988)

		Percentage of Change (1983–1988)
Visits:[a][b]		
	Ambulatory Surgery[c]	115% Increase
	Emergency Department	9% Increase
	Organized Outpatient Department[d]	19% Increase
	Other Outpatient Service[e]	23% Increase
Programs:[f]		
	Ambulatory Surgery[g]	5% Increase
	Emergency Departments	3% Decrease
	Organized Outpatient Departments	47% Increase
	Other Outpatient Services	
	Health Promotion	91% Increase
	Home Care	115% Increase
	Hospice	48% Increase
	Rehabilitation	20% Increase
	Psychiatry	16% Increase
	Chemical Dependency	37% Increase

[a]AHA annual survey.
[b]Visits for 1988 used to obtain Percentage of Change were projected figures, Division of Ambulatory Care and Health Promotion.
[c]Surgical services provided to patients who do not remain in the hospital overnight.
[d]Visits by patients who are not lodged in the hospital while receiving medical, dental, or other services. Each appearance by an outpatient to each unit of the hospital counts as one outpatient visit.
[e]Refers to outpatient therapy and treatment visits, ancillary service visits, and all other forms of outpatient care not previously defined; also includes ambulatory surgery visits.
[f] AHA hospital statistics; approximately 90% of hospitals reported for each year.
[g]Information not reported until 1983.

Source: Adapted with permission from "Transition in Ambulatory Care" by Diane M. Howard, Director, Division of Ambulatory Care and Health Promotion, American Hospital Association, from presentation to the Joint Commission on Accreditation of Healthcare Organizations, August 19, 1990.

- group practices
- armed services programs
- cardiac catheterization centers
- Native American health service centers
- primary care centers
- urgent/emergency care centers

For the purpose of this discussion, this author includes health maintenance and related managed care organizations, both staff and independent practice models.

As the volume and complexity of health care provided in ambulatory settings increase, external bodies that evaluate and pay for care delivered in these settings are devoting increasing attention not only to the cost, but also to the quality of the care provided. And an expectation of continuity between and among inpatient and outpatient systems of care is beginning to develop. However, expectations are not as well defined as they are for inpatient services where Joint Commission accreditation has been an expectation for over two decades. The message is that if ambulatory care professionals don't lead or actively participate in deciding how quality will be defined and monitored in our practice settings, we could easily find ourselves living with unrealistic expectations and monitoring procedures provided to us by decision makers unfamiliar with the characteristics of ambulatory care.

KEY ISSUES IN AMBULATORY CARE

Key issues that affect the ability to monitor and evaluate the quality of care in an ambulatory setting relate to

- characteristics of care in the ambulatory setting
- quality assurance issues in ambulatory settings

Relevant Characteristics of Ambulatory Care

One of the most apparent relevant characteristics of ambulatory care is patient control versus provider control. Patients decide when they will come in, whether they will comply with self-care directions, and whether they will seek care elsewhere if dissatisfied. They may mix professional regimens with home/folk medicine regimens. They may not view follow-up and preventive care visits with the same enthusiasm as we do, especially if they must pay for them out of pocket. Conserving gas money or time off work may take priority over blood pressure checks or post–otitis media re-examination.

A related issue is what some refer to as the "art of care." The art of care could be described as the ability to learn the key realities of patients' life situations, to effectively educate patients/family members about actual or potential health problems, to involve them in development of self-care plans that recognize the key realities, and, finally, to motivate patients to follow through. The burden of follow-through is on the patient in ambulatory care. Without a trust exchange of information and perceptions, follow-through and positive outcomes are jeopardized.

Another characteristic of ambulatory care is that frequently an ambulatory medical visit may not result in a clear-cut medical diagnosis. In contrast, there usually is a definite plan as to what the results of a hospitalization should be, with some integration of services received there.

The scope of services offered in ambulatory settings varies widely from single or small partner traditional physician practices offering basic "primary care" to large multidisciplinary and/or multispecialty centers. Whether professional nurses are present and, if so, what roles they play in ambulatory settings vary widely also.

Fragmentation is another relevant characteristic of ambulatory care. Services for multiple problems may be obtained from multiple sources without coordination. How well are outcomes monitored? Does the abnormal pap smear get followed up? Does an active problem list exist anywhere that summarizes a patient's medical and psychosocial problems that impact on his/her level of health? Medical specialization and reimbursement systems that have typically paid for "process" services without regard to coordination or "health of the patient" outcomes provide a legacy major payers are deciding they can no longer afford.

Lack of normative information on which to base judgments is another characteristic of ambulatory settings. Ambulatory medical records are often inconsistent in format and content. Problem or summary lists are difficult to implement. Other documentation systems often are manually done and difficult to maintain. How many ambulatory centers track the follow-up of abnormal pap smear results they receive or consistently monitor availability of lab and x-ray reports? As computerization becomes more realistic to implement in ambulatory settings and as expectations of quality documentation increase, improvement in the collection and processing of data is a growing possibility and priority.

In summary, ambulatory settings are diverse, and the issues that impact on the health of the patient are complex.

Ambulatory Quality Assurance Issues

The characteristics of ambulatory centers as a category raise the following questions in relation to quality assurance (QA):

- How do we define quality?
- How and what should we monitor?
- When is a deficiency a problem?
- Why aren't problems solved?

How Do We Define Quality?

The health care literature provides consistent definition of quality. In the community health centers operated by Methodist Hospital of Indiana, Inc., we have adapted and adopted a 1974 Institute of Medicine policy statement in which the primary goal of a QA system was proposed to be "health care that effectively betters the health status and satisfaction of the population, within the resources that society and individuals have chosen to spend for that care" (Institute of Medicine, 1974).

This definition encompasses dimensions of quality that can be used in developing a quality ambulatory care program. It can be used to focus on what quality really is in developing a structure to evaluate the quality of our program. Thus, both the development of the ambulatory care program and the evaluation (quality assurance) of that program can be based on the dimensions of quality included in this definition. This definition focuses on evidence of improvement, not necessarily cure; it recognizes patient perception as an important part of evaluation; and it recognizes the reality of limited resources with which to accomplish improvement.

Other terms are used inconsistently in health care quality assurance. For clarity, *quality assurance* is being defined as a structured and comprehensive system to monitor and evaluate the entire ambulatory clinical care program and to resolve deficiencies in that care when discovered. Other key terms that are defined inconsistently in the QA arena are *standard, indicator, criterion,* and *threshold*. These terms are used here as follows:

- *Standard:* performance expectation for a given indicator, as determined by the individual ambulatory organization
- *Indicator:* what is looked at to determine how well the organization is doing on an aspect of care
- *Criterion:* not used
- *Threshold:* Expectation of how close to meeting a standard an organization's performance must come; performance below (or above, in the case of negative performance) the threshold requires evaluation and problem-solving efforts to improve the quality and/or appropriateness of care
- *Quality Improvement Plan (QIP) Level:* a term used in the AMBUQUAL® quality assurance and quality management system described later; similar to the term *threshold* in that it is a numerical level of performance on a particular indicator below which problem evaluation and problem-solving efforts are initiated by an organization.

The meanings assigned to these key words in this chapter are compared in Figure 7-1 to meanings assigned in the writings of Avedis Donabedian and in Joint Commission publications.

Donabedian	JCAHO	AMBUQUAL®
Aspect	Aspect	Aspect
Indicator	Indicator	Indicator
Criterion		Standard
Standard	Threshold	QIP Level

Figure 7-1 Key Quality Assurance Terms. *Source:* Courtesy of Dale S. Benson, MD, Director of Ambulatory Care Services, Methodist Hospital of Indiana, Inc., Indianapolis, IN.

Definitions from Donabedian, A. (1987, September) *A Primer of Quality Assurance and Monitoring in Medical Care.* Paper presented at the Conference on Law Practice Quality Evaluation: An Appraisal of Peer Review and Other Measures to Enhance Professional Performance (sponsored by the American Law Institute and the American Bar Association, Committee on Continuing Professional Education), Williamsburg, VA; Benson, D.S. & Miller, J.A., (1989). *AMBUQUAL®: An ambulatory quality assurance and quality management system,* Indianapolis: Methodist Hospital of Indiana, Inc.; Joint Commission on Accreditation of Healthcare Organizations. (1990). *The Joint Commission 1990 Ambulatory Health care standards manual.* Chicago: Author.

How and What Should We Monitor?

What is monitoring? The key is to understand what monitoring means. *Monitoring* means to look at something on an ongoing basis. *Ongoing* means that one looks at something once a day, or once a week, or once a month, or once a quarter, or once a year. How often one looks at it depends on how important it is.

Thus, to monitor and evaluate a clinical care program, one must identify important areas of the program and then look at these areas on an ongoing basis. When you look at these areas, then the evaluation activity occurs. *Evaluation* is simply making a judgment about how well the organization is performing in the area being monitored.

Organizations can approach quality assurance by focusing on one discipline, such as nursing, or they can take a multidisciplinary approach. Because the numbers for individual disciplines are often small in ambulatory settings, a multidisciplinary approach to quality assurance often makes more sense. Two multidisciplinary approaches will be described: A generic and open-ended approach will be outlined here; AMBUQUAL®, a flexible, but structured, approach will be discussed later in the chapter.

Choosing what to monitor is the place to start in setting up the monitoring phase of an ambulatory QA program. Ambulatory organizations currently have a great deal of flexibility in deciding for themselves what to monitor. This is a fundamentally important decision and one that can profoundly impact on the success of the program. Following is a functional, three-step suggestion for how to choose what to monitor.

In the first step, define the clinical program (scope). Because it is essential that important phases of the program are not missing, the place to start is by defining what the clinical program really includes. What kind of approach can be used to ensure that important parts of the clinical program are not being left out of the QA activity? Ask questions such as these:

- What do physicians do in this setting?
- What do dentists do in this setting?
- What do nurses do in this setting?
- What about lab, or pharmacy, or x-ray?
- What is the scope of services that are provided for patients in this setting?

It is useful to keep in mind that the purpose of quality assurance is the improved health of your patients. Therefore, QA activities should focus on clinical issues that have potential to impact on patient well-being. Energy may be wasted on issues that have no potential to improve your patient's health.

The second step is to identify important aspects of the clinical care program. Once the spectrum or scope of the clinical care program has been defined, identify the most important components to monitor. High-volume, high-risk, or problem prone and potentially inappropriate activities are logical selections.

The third step in deciding what to monitor is to specify what component(s) of an important aspect will be monitored—in other words, to identify indicators.

An important monitoring strategy in ambulatory care is to start simple and to choose only a few indicators to monitor when beginning a QA program (Benson & Townes, 1990). The program can expand gradually as experience in monitoring grows. Accrediting-body surveyors expect to see evidence that monitoring is occurring. Some monitoring is better than none. An overzealous beginning may result in system burnout—so start simple. It is important, however, to point out that the flexibility to start simple may not be possible much longer in ambulatory organizations. Some reimbursement arrangements may have already imposed specific monitoring expectations on organizations, a phenomenon quite familiar to hospitals and some managed-care organizations.

After deciding what to monitor, two implementation decisions need to be made before beginning an ambulatory care monitoring program. For each indicator to be monitored, decide (1) how frequently it will be looked at and (2) where and how the needed data will be obtained.

Many indicators need to be monitored only once a year. For instance, in order to assure that provider credentials remain current and complete, once a year is often enough to take a look. Other indicators may need to be monitored more frequently. A quarterly review of patient satisfaction may be appropriate.

Once the "what" and "when" questions of indicator monitoring have been answered, the monitoring agendas for a calendar year of QA meetings can be written.

Where data will come from is a major issue in the monitoring process. Here, again, it is important to remember the "keep it simple" concept.

If the standard is a quantitative one, and if the data are available, then it is easy for the QA committee to compare the data to the standard. For example, assume documentation is available on current licenses for 90 percent of the licensed personnel in the organization. The threshold is 100 percent, and 90 percent is less than 100 percent. Therefore, problem-solving activities should be initiated.

If the standard is qualitative, then the judgment of the QA committee becomes more important and more difficult. This judgment draws on the observations and experience of the committee members. For instance, to monitor whether or not you have a patient grievance procedure that works, the QA committee members can provide the data (observation and experience input) needed.

Four questions will help the QA committee make a judgment regarding the performance of its ambulatory care center in relation to a qualitative (non-quantitative) standard.

1. Is this a clinical care problem? The committee must make the judgment that this problem has the potential to directly impact on the health of the patient.
2. Is this a prevalent problem? The committee must agree that this problem occurs frequently enough that it must be solved or that it is of such significance that all effort must be taken to be certain that it never happens again.
3. Is there a solution to this problem? Various constraints may lead to a realistic decision that this problem cannot be solved. In that case, invest energy working on something else.
4. Is the benefit to the patient worth the cost or effort of solving the problem?

If the answer to each of these questions is "yes," the QA committee should designate an official QA problem. The remainder of the problem resolution activity then occurs (Benson & Miller, 1988).

When Is a Deficiency a Problem?

To evaluate simply requires the QA committee to make a judgment regarding how well the organization is performing on any particular indicator. Before the QA committee can make this judgment, one critical step needs to be taken: to define the standard of the organization for each indicator that is to be monitored. Without a predetermined standard, it is impossible for the QA committee to make a judgment.

An example of standard setting could relate to an indicator that monitors diastolic blood pressure control in hypertensive patients. The standard might be that hypertension patients should have a diastolic pressure below 95 after six months of treatment. Perhaps the threshold is set at 90 percent, meaning that 90 percent of the charts sampled for hypertensive patients who have been under treatment at least six months show documentation of a diastolic pressure of 95 or below. Once the standard has been defined and the threshold set, the evaluation phase of monitoring becomes quite simple. The QA committee need only compare the actual performance of your organization (from the audit data) against the predetermined standard and threshold of the organization.

It is important for an organization to establish its own standards. The professional staff should be involved in their development because this will increase the chances that they will buy into quality assurance. We typically are more willing to have our performance evaluated against standards that we helped set as opposed to the arbitrary application of somebody else's standards to us.

It is also important that an organization's standards be clinically valid. This means that they should be compatible with current knowledge and expertise as well as with the practice realities of the individual setting. A good rule of thumb is that a clinically valid standard will make sense to outside professionals familiar with the setting. If there is confidence that a standard will seem reasonable to other professional people, then it is probably a clinically valid standard.

The composition of the QA committee should be multidisciplinary and should emphasize involvement of the people delivering the care. This approach suggests representation that includes all those employee groups that support the delivery of patient care: reception/cashier, medical assistant, and medical records people, as well as care providers such as physicians, nurses, and social workers. Including front line care givers on the QA committee and rotating people from clinical or support service job categories on and off the QA committee provide multiple perspectives that can result in a clearer picture of where systems problems exist. It also helps get more people involved and increases their knowledge about the QA program. The clinical and administrative leadership personnel in the ambulatory organization should be responsible for developing the QA program and setting standards. In small ambulatory organizations, some members of the QA committee probably will be part of the clinical or administrative leadership. However, conducting the standard and threshold setting process up front, separate from the evaluation, helps maintain the integrity of the evaluation process even if nearly the same group is making evaluation judgments.

Why Aren't Problems Solved?

Common reasons why quality-related ambulatory problems are not solved include the following:

- The problem is poorly defined.
- No allowance is made for human error.
- Responsibility for solving the problem is unclear.
- The person(s) responsible do not accept the problem or do not consider it a priority.
- The organization expects the QA committee to solve all quality-related problems.
- The person(s) responsible do not have sufficient clout or resources to fix the problem.
- The organization does not support resolution of quality-related problems from the highest level.
- No deadline is set.
- No follow-up monitoring is carried out.

Three fundamental problem-solving principles guide the Methodist Hospital approach to ambulatory quality assurance. The first is that the QA committee does not solve problems. The role of the QA committee is simply to monitor and evaluate the important aspects of clinical care in the organization and refer any potential problems discovered to the administrative or clinical management structure of the organization for problem-solving activity.

The second priniciple is that quality-related problems should be identified and solved at the level where the problem occurs. The ambulatory center should be organized so that physicians can identify and solve their problems, nurses can identify and solve their problems, the lab can identify and solve its problems, and so on. None of these groups should be dependent on the QA committee to identify and solve quality-related problems. In fact, such quality-related problems should be identified and solved regardless of whether or not a QA program even exists. The QA program becomes important if, during monitoring and evaluation, it is discovered that a problem that should have been identified and solved at its own level has "slipped through the cracks."

The third principle is that the ultimate mission of quality assurance is to improve human performance. It is the interface between the nurse or the physician and the patient where quality really resides. In quality assurance, we want to improve the level of performance of the provider in order to raise the level of quality in that interface. When the provider performance is inadequate, it is in the vast majority of cases the result of a poorly functioning system. Fixing the system leads to a higher level of performance at the interface. Therefore, a QA program should monitor and evaluate systems as well as individual performance within these systems. In evaluating the effectiveness of a QA program, there must be evidence that it is more than a mechanical exercise. The end result of QA activities should be better service to the patient (Benson & Van Osdol, 1990).

THE AMBUQUAL® APPROACH

A comprehensive and balanced approach to conducting patient care–focused QA activities in ambulatory settings has been developed under the leadership of Dale S. Benson MD, through the Ambulatory Care Services department at Methodist Hospital of Indiana, Inc., and the Community Health Network of Indianapolis. The approach, a system called AMBUQUAL, is computer assisted and has the unique ability to quantify the quality of care using a weighted scoring system (Benson & Miller, 1989). This QA system focuses on the monitoring, evaluation, problem identification, and problem resolution activities that have the potential to impact on the health of patients in the ambulatory setting. The initial development of this system was partially supported by a grant from Region V, U.S. Department of Health and Human Services.

The Structure

The AMBUQUAL system is based on ten parameters of care, perspectives from which to view an ambulatory care program. These parameters are comparable to the 12 different perspectives from which a cardiogram views the heart in that they provide a view of the ambulatory care program from ten different perspectives. Together, these ten parameters provide a comprehensive picture of the quality of any given ambulatory clinical program and constitute the scope of the ambulatory QA program in centers monitoring and evaluating services using the AMBU-QUAL system (Benson, Gartner, Anderson, Schweer, & Kirchgessner, 1987). The ten parameters are

- provider staff performance
- support staff performance
- continuity of care
- medical records system
- patient risk minimization
- patient satisfaction
- patient compliance
- accessibility
- appropriateness of service
- cost of services

AMBUQUAL divides each parameter into four logical areas, which are called *aspects of care*. The 40 resulting ambulatory aspects of care, considered applicable in any ambulatory setting, focus on clinical activities or concerns that can impact on the health of the patient. They include activities or concerns that involve a high volume of patients, that entail a high risk for patients, that are problem prone and are potentially inappropriate.

For each aspect of care, AMBUQUAL defines from one to seven indicators of care, with the potential for up to ten. These indicators address structure, process, and outcome issues common to ambulatory care. Each indicator has its own clinically valid standard and has the potential to impact on the health of the patient. Some of the indicators are considered applicable in any ambulatory care setting and are, therefore, designated as *fundamental indicators*, with the expectation they will be monitored by the system's users. Other indicators are considered site specific and can be eliminated, revised, or replaced with others as judged appropriate by members of the user organization. The indicator standards provided are generic in nature, so specific organizations have the flexibility to adapt them where necessary. Thresholds for problem evaluation and resolution activity are determined by members of the user organization. A structured problem resolution process defines responsibility ultimately up to the governing body level to assure that quality-related problems are addressed.

Structure Indicators

An example of a parameter along with a related aspect and structural indicator follows:

> *Parameter:* Provider staff performance
> *Aspect:* Credentials
> *Indicator:* Licensure

Standard: Licensure required by the state is current and verified for all applicable provider staff.
Data Source: Personnel folder

Process Indicators

An example of a parameter along with a related aspect and process indicator follows:

Parameter: Patient compliance
Aspect: Understanding of health care plan
Indicator: Patient education regarding medications and therapies
Standard: All patients who start new medications or therapies should receive education specific to these new medications or therapies.

Outcome Indicators

Efforts to monitor outcomes focus currently on the patient satisfaction and patient compliance parameters and look at patient perception. Examples of parameters along with related aspects and outcome indicators follow:

Parameter: Patient satisfaction
Aspect: Satisfaction with ambulatory care center
Indicator: Waiting time
Standard: Patients indicate satisfaction with the waiting time.

Parameter: Patient compliance
Aspect: Compliance with health care plan
Indicator: Treatment plan
Standard: Patients state they complied with their most recent treatment plan.

Note: This indicator is preceded by indicators that monitor structure and process issues that relate to ensuring that patients participate in treatment plan development and that they are provided with information they would need to comply with the plan.

Also included are indicators that monitor short-term negative *systems outcomes*. Two examples follow:

Parameter: Patient risk minimization
Aspect: Patient safety
Indicator: Patient incident report trending

Standard: Incidents reported are summarized by type at least annually. Reports are reviewed for significant trends, and problem areas are addressed.

Note: This is an approach to controlling negative outcomes of patients' presence in the facility.

Parameter: Accessibility
Aspect: Ease/timeliness of access to professional advice
Indicator: Telephone access during clinic hours
    Standard: Patients report that they are able to talk to a member of the provider staff via telephone on the same day advice is sought.

The AMBUQUAL system is structured to facilitate ongoing cyclical review of all components (approximately 150 indicators). To evaluate performance in relation to indicator standards, data are needed, and data source development is a major task. Some data may be available in the ambulatory setting, but may not be retrievable in a meaningful form. AMBUQUAL implementation is, therefore, structured in three graduated levels. This allows the user organization to start monitoring only a few indicators at a time, adding more indicators in later cycles. Thus, managers and QA committee members can become familiar with the system and set up sources of data gradually.

Application

AMBUQUAL provides a monitoring, evaluation, and problem identification/resolution structure that is applicable, with minor alterations, in most ambulatory settings. Settings where implementation is occurring are private physician group practices, group model HMOs, hospital-based ambulatory centers, community health centers, and a regional cancer center.

The Scoring Component

AMBUQUAL offers a computer-assisted scoring component that allows an ambulatory care center to monitor its quality of care performance over time by monitoring and comparing one number—the *program quality index* (PQI). Figure 7-2 portrays the flow of data in the form of scores leading to the PQI; Figure 7-3 portrays the path of scores from a specific indicator to the PQI summary score.

The scoring system assigns weights to each indicator, aspect, and parameter according to expert perception of their importance to quality of care. For example,

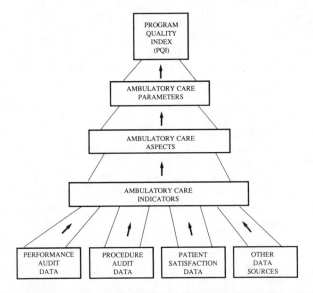

Figure 7-2 AMBUQUAL®: A Quantitative Approach to Measuring the Quality of Ambulatory Care. *Source:* Courtesy of Methodist Hospital of Indiana, Inc., Indianapolis, IN.

provider performance is weighted more heavily than is accessibility of services. Joint Commission ambulatory surveyors provided expert input into the assignment of parameter weights (Anderson et al., 1989). The scoring system generates a score between 0 and 100 at the indicator, aspect, parameter, and PQI levels. Scores at the indicator level are obtained by one of two processes: (1) an objective score, usually a percentage for data compliance with the standard, or (2) a score generated from a process in which the QA committee judges the level of standard fulfillment and the probable impact of deficiencies on patient care.

An example of a computer-generated PQI summary score report is shown in Table 7-2; a computer-generated parameter score report (patient compliance) is shown in Table 7-3. The computer software that supports the AMBUQUAL system can generate summary and parameter reports of the organization's quantitative level of quality at any point in time.

Credibility Concerns

The task force that developed AMBUQUAL has striven to assure compliance with Joint Commission Standards for Ambulatory Care. To date, five ambulatory centers have successfully undergone Joint Commission survey subsequent to

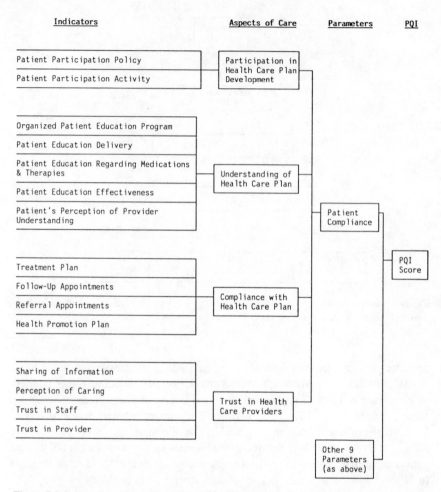

Figure 7-3 Patient Compliance Example—AMBUQUAL® system. *Source:* Courtesy of Methodist Hospital of Indiana, Inc., Indianapolis, IN.

implementing AMBUQUAL. In each case, the rating of the center's QA program supports the validity of AMBUQUAL as an ambulatory QA system.

Multidisciplinary Scope

AMBUQUAL's structure supports a multidisciplinary approach to quality assurance in the ambulatory setting. Each primary care organization must define its provider group; how it does so depends on the roles various disciplines assume

Table 7-2 Program Quality Index Summary Score Report

AMBUQUAL—PROGRAM QUALITY INDEX (PQI)
Super Center USA 12-22-90

Parameter	Score	Weight	Description
1	62	1.92	Provider Staff Performance
2	84	1.11	Support Staff Performance
3	73	0.90	Continuity of Care
4	81	0.68	Medical Records System
5	64	0.70	Patient Risk Minimization
6	92	0.59	Patient Satisfaction
7	76	1.25	Patient Compliance
8	86	0.91	Accessibility
9	63	1.39	Appropriateness of Service
10	87	0.54	Cost of Services

Program Quality Index = 74

Source: Courtesy of Dale S. Benson, MD, Methodist Hospital of Indiana, Inc., Indianapolis, IN.

within that organization. Once provider groups are defined, credentials, current competence, and clinical performance are aspects monitored for each provider group. Peer performance review is an expectation of each provider group, with results evaluated at the individual and group levels.

Although there are advantages to a multidisciplinary approach to quality assurance, there are also potential problems that can become disadvantages. This is particularly true in the ambulatory setting. Reimbursement drives what happens in health care delivery. In ambulatory care, current reimbursement is physician directed and controlled, with only rare exceptions (such as grant-funded services and demonstration projects). Further, currently reimbursable ambulatory services are primarily ''process'' services. There is no direct link between reimbursement and evidence of appropriateness, quality of the process, or evidence of expected outcomes. In this environment, the worth of the physician's time and billable services easily takes precedence over what other disciplines can contribute independently to the health of the patient, assuming other disciplines are even part of the provider team. In Figure 7-4, Schroeder presents a comparison between single discipline and multidisciplinary approaches to quality assurance that highlights the potential problems of multidisciplinary quality assurance.

NURSING QA ISSUES SPECIFIC TO THE AMBULATORY SETTING

The presence of professional nurses is not a given in the ambulatory setting, a major difference from the hospital inpatient setting. The presence of professional

Table 7-3 Patient Compliance Parameter Score Report

AMBUQUAL—PROGRAM QUALITY INDEX (PQI)
Super Center USA 12-22-90

	Last Update	Score	Weight	Description
Parameter 7		76	1.25	Patient Compliance
Aspect A		**30**	**0.60**	**Patient participation in health care plan development**
7.A.1	1/29/88	100	0.60	Patient participation policy
7.A.2	4/22/87	0	1.40	Patient participation activity
Aspect B		**95**	**1.30**	**Understanding of health care plan**
7.B.1	1/29/88	100	1.00	Organized patient education program
7.B.2	2/25/88	96	1.00	Patient education delivery
7.B.3	2/25/88	91	1.00	Patient education re: meds and therapies
7.B.4	2/25/88	95	1.00	Patient education effectiveness
7.B.5	2/25/88	96	1.00	Patient understanding of provider
7.B.6	2/25/88	94	1.00	Patient perception of provider understanding
Aspect C		**66**	**1.30**	**Compliance with health care plan**
7.C.1	2/25/88	93	1.10	Treatment plan
7.C.2	3/25/88	100	1.10	Follow-up appointments
7.C.3	2/25/88	0	0.90	Referral appointments
7.C.4	2/25/88	56	0.90	Health promotion plan
Aspect D		**95**	**0.80**	**Trust in health care providers**
7.D.1	2/25/88	94	0.80	Sharing of information
7.D.2	2/25/88	94	1.30	Perception of caring
7.D.3	2/25/88	95	0.80	Trust in staff
7.D.4	2/25/88	98	1.10	Trust in provider

Source: Courtesy of Dale S. Benson, MD, Methodist Hospital of Indiana, Inc., Indianapolis, IN.

nursing practice in the ambulatory setting is most certainly not a given. Historically, major third-party payers reimburse physicians for medical diagnosis– and treatment–related services. In some ambulatory settings, nurse practitioners or nurse clinicians have been able to gain acceptance as capable and efficient "physician extenders" or are valued for their patient education and case management skills. However, with rare exceptions, they have remained a "cost," instead of a "revenue generator," in the ambulatory reimbursement system. This role makes them extremely vulnerable to extinction as providers during any budgetary review based on traditional billing/revenue generation systems. One step toward greater monetary value was passed by the U.S. Congress in December 1989. This legislation provides for direct payment from Medicaid to certified pediatric and family nurse practitioners (NPs) for services they provide within the scope of state law, regardless of whether the NP is supervised by or associated with a physician

	Single Discipline	Multidisciplinary
Focus of QA	Practice of profession	Clients/families
Accountability/ boundaries of practice	Assumed	Blurred—clear negotiation necessary
Interdisciplinary relationships necessary	None	Professional, trusting that all are working toward good of the client/family
Degree of focus on each discipline	Complete	Relatively easy to omit involvement of a group
Responsibility for carrying out the work of QA	Often appointed or shared	Often assumed, based on perceived authority, worth of time
Perceived rationale for difficulty in process	Joint Commission	Interpersonal/ interdisciplinary conflicts

Figure 7-4 Multidisciplinary Quality Assurance. *Source:* Courtesy of Patricia Schroeder, Independent Nursing Quality Consultant, Thiensville, WI.

(Vanderbilt, 1990). This means reimbursement can be paid by Medicaid directly to the nurse practitioner, but only for those services Medicaid will reimburse and, of these services, only for ones these providers may provide *independently* (i.e., without physician supervision). An example would be well child examinations (M.W. Vanderbilt, personal communication, January 18, 1990).

When professional nurses are present in the ambulatory setting, they often are there in a center operations management role, rather than in a direct practice role. In this role, emphasis is on efficient management of a system that supports the delivery of services by others. In such a role, there is neither authority nor accountability for direct independent services to the patient. Consequently, nurse manager involvement in direct services may be unofficial and without recognized independent value or evaluation in the QA system.

In those ambulatory settings where professional nursing practice occurs, can AMBUQUAL monitor and evaluate that nursing practice? AMBUQUAL does not define which provider discipline delivers services. But AMBUQUAL does, through the expectation of peer review, accommodate the documentation of the nursing process, so that not only the services delivered but also the contexts in which the nurse delivers the service are described. The model for nursing quality assurance described by Hastings (1987) provides an approach to the nursing peer review component of the provider clinical performance audit. AMBUQUAL aspects and indicators of care for which nurses possess particular concern and skills are specifically monitored in AMBUQUAL. These include patient participation in health care plan development, patient understanding of the health care plan, appropriateness of services, and accessibility of services, as well as continuity of care issues.

Professional nurses can often be found assuming one of two roles in ambulatory quality assurance. One QA role is as coordinator of the program that monitors and evaluates organizational systems and the practice of other disciplines, primarily physicians, within those systems. As expectations for and the value of quality assurance increase in the ambulatory setting, the demand for nurses to fill this coordinator role may increase. However, other disciplines, such as medical records and management information specialists, may compete successfully for this role.

Another QA role professional nurses may assume is that of provider involved in peer review for the purpose of identifying opportunities to improve. This role presumes the presence of professional nursing practice as a medical extender, in a collaborative role, or, in those instances where nurses have been able to establish it, in independent practice. Each of these practice roles dictates a different monitoring approach. In collaborative and medical extender roles, the nurse's practice would be monitored in a multidisciplinary model. However, in the medical extender role, the nurse would be monitored against protocols of practice supervised by a physician. In the collaborative role, there would be both medical and nursing monitors. Nurses in independent practice could take a "single discipline" approach to quality assurance.

CONCLUSION

The dynamics of the ambulatory setting are quite different from those of the hospital inpatient setting, where the majority of nurses have historically practiced. Patients control their entry and may judge entry and quality decisions using a very different value system and standards than do health care professionals. Services delivered and reimbursed in the ambulatory setting have traditionally been medical diagnosis and treatment at the primary and specialty levels. Quality assurance has not been an expectation or a priority. However, changes in reimbursement policy are creating a rapid increase in the volume and complexity of services delivered in the ambulatory setting. Major payers are beginning to ask for evidence of quality, especially as it relates to appropriateness and efficiency. This increases the interest of ambulatory care organizations in accreditation and quality assurance. The continuity of care that patients receive across the continuum of inpatient, ambulatory, and home care services becomes an expectation when reimbursement moves from fee for medical units of service to case management models with outcome monitoring, a developing focus.

The ambulatory care environment is undergoing great change. Professional nursing has not played a strong role in the ambulatory care environment, but nursing practice and nurses have much to offer efficient, comprehensive care delivery and care evaluation in the ambulatory setting. New reimbursement systems pose the potential for reward for preventive care, early assessment and problem identification, patient education, and case management. Professional nurses are well qualified to provide these skills at a competitive price. At this time, there is a critical need for organized nursing to demonstrate this value in the form of evidence and political pressure. Professional nurses need to work through their professional organizations' political and public policy coalitions to inform and lobby. This effort should target health policy boards and other forums from the institutional level to the national legislative and regulatory levels. It should also target private sector payer and accreditation groups. Patient-focused QA systems can support professional nursing in these efforts in ambulatory as well as other settings.

REFERENCES

Anderson, J.G., Benson, D.S., Schweer, H.M., Gartner, C.G., & Jay, S.J. (1989). Ambuqual: A computer-supported system for the measurement and evaluation of quality in ambulatory care settings. *Journal of Ambulatory Care Management, 12,* 27–37.

Benson, D.S., Gartner, C.G., Anderson, J.G., Schweer, H.M., & Kirchgessner, R.L. (1987). The ambulatory care parameter: A structured approach to quality assurance in the ambulatory care setting. *Quality Review Bulletin, 13,* 51–55.

Benson, D.S., & Miller, J.M. (1988). *Quality assurance for primary care centers.* Indianapolis: Methodist Hospital of Indiana, Inc.

Benson, D.S., & Miller, J.A. (1989). *Ambuqual®: An ambulatory quality assurance and quality management system.* Indianapolis: Methodist Hospital of Indiana, Inc.

Benson, D.S., & Townes, P.G. (1990). *Excellence in ambulatory care: A practical guide to developing effective quality assurance programs.* San Franciso: Jossey Bass.

Benson, D.S., & Van Osdol, W.R. (1990). *Quality audit systems for primary care centers* (2nd ed.). Indianapolis: Methodist Hospital of Indiana, Inc.

Donabedian, A. (1987, September). *A primer of quality assurance and monitoring in medical care.* Paper presented at the Conference on Law Practice Quality Evaluation: An Appraisal of Peer Review and other Measures To Enhance Professional Performance (sponsored by the American Law Institute and the American Bar Association, Committee on Continuing Professional Education), Williamsburg, VA.

Hastings, C. (1987). Measuring quality in ambulatory care nursing. *Journal of Nursing Administration, 12,* 12–21.

Institute of Medicine. (1974). *Advancing the quality of health care: Key issues and fundamental principles.* Washington, DC: National Academy of Sciences, 1–2.

Joint Commission on Accreditation of Healthcare Organizations. (1990). *Joint Commission 1990 ambulatory health care standards manual.* Chicago: Author.

Vanderbilt, M. (1990). Budget provisions are victory: Advanced practice nurses to benefit. *American Nurse, 1,* 17.

8

Monitoring Practice: A Home Care Example

Claire Meisenheimer, PhD, RN, CNAA, Associate Professor, University of
Wisconsin, College of Nursing, Graduate Program, Oshkosh, Wisconsin

The inevitable revolution in the way health care services will be delivered in the
next decade is already having far-reaching economic and social impact on consumers, providers, third-party payers, regulators, and policy makers alike. Science, a major revolutionary force, is delivering biomedical breakthroughs that
hold the promise of remarkable cures for illness and the threat of unacceptable
causes of death. Optimism about medicine's ability to prolong life over the next
50 years has been projected in a study by the University of California and the
National Institute of Aging: "The over 65 population in the United States may
jump to 87 million, or one-quarter of the entire U.S. population by the year
2040—20 million people more than the Census Bureau has projected and 3 times
the current level" (Elderly Health, 1988). The graying of America is resulting
from a burgeoning elderly population that consumes the most expensive high-tech
medicine; this population also tests our capacity to provide adequate medical and
nursing care for the growing numbers experiencing normal aging associated with
chronic illness and disability. If current rates of disability persist, it is estimated
that by the year 2000, over 15 million older Americans will suffer from chronic
disease that will limit their daily activities, a 50 percent increase over 1980
(Spiegel, 1987).

Since 1980, health costs have soared at a rate far exceeding that of inflation and
are currently approaching 12 percent of the gross national product (GNP). Regulatory controls by the federal and state governments, the largest purchasers of
health services, are reflected in the reimbursement of Medicare and Medicaid
patients for services provided at rates far below health agency costs, while the
monitoring of over- and underutilization of services continues. Professional
review organizations (PROs), the deemed overseers of medical care quality under
Medicare, are working closely with the Health Care Financing Administration
(HCFA) to determine measures of quality in "intervening care" other than
traditional indicators, such as mortality rates. Other fiscal intermediaries, such as

Blue Cross and Blue Shield and other employer groups, are examining deviations from accepted norms and noting HCFA benchmarks that may create standards that set the pace for the private and public sectors alike.

Accrediting bodies, such as the Joint Commission on Accreditation of Healthcare Organizations, have revised their approach (1) to focus quality review on clinical performance measures and outcomes, adjusted for the severity of patient illness, and (2) to impose sanctions (including "conditional accreditation") on organizations that do not comply. The issue is no longer one of "whether an organization can provide care," but one of "whether an organization provides high-quality care."

The issues of access, cost, and quality are demanding new paradigms that can more efficaciously solve the problems of the current health care system. While the model for acute care is the predominate model for care in the United States, the future of health care demands us to view the *home* as the center of care, and that requires a new health care delivery paradigm.

The home has always been the place where families have cared for their members; it is a component on the illness-wellness continuum that is "assumed." Its evolution, however, as examined by Stanhope (1989), has provided consumers, professionals, legislators, and payers with not only numerous opportunities, but new concerns as well (U.S. Congress, 1986). The proliferation of home care agencies from 208 in 1961 to a $10 billion industry comprising an estimated 12,000 to 14,000 provider agencies in 1988 (Moore, 1988), has resulted in an expanded range of care and increased types of services.

The wide array of medical and nonmedical services designed to manage all needs from acute episodic care needs to sustaining home care needs for functionally impaired individuals is frequently divided into (1) health-related care, provided by medical and nursing personnel, and (2) personal care including assistance with basic activities of daily living (ADLs), provided by assistants and other care workers and supervised by professionals. Case management has emerged as a critical issue as providers attempt to coordinate existing service delivery systems with the various funding sources. While increasing clients' access to care and services, coordinating services provided by multiple agencies, and ensuring that services are allocated efficiently and equitably, the overriding issue is, What is quality in home care, and what are the best ways of monitoring and evaluating that delivery system?

QUALITY ASSURANCE ISSUES IN HOME CARE

Assuring quality care to the frail and dependent clients who are hidden in their homes away from public view is particularly difficult when there are no universally established standards for quality in home care. There is also no consensus on what constitutes quality among and between the various participant groups. Due to inadequate and inconsistent external regulation and monitoring, generic, systematic descriptions of quality problems in home care are not currently available. Such sources as *The "Black Box" of Home Care Quality* (U.S. Congress, 1986), Applebaum and Christianson (1988), and Applebaum and Wilson (1988) have highlighted several factors that compromise home care quality: caregiver abuse, neglect, exploitation, absenteeism, and tardiness; failure to complete assigned caregiving tasks, including the following of medical orders; inappropriate matching of home care personnel to clients' needs; and the usage of technological equipment that in previous times had been seen only in intensive care units.

While individual horror stories have been identified in the news media, in various legislative reports, and in expert testimony on home care (U.S. Congress, 1985), today's consumers—our clients and families—are more sophisticated, are asking questions, and are involved in their care. Caregivers are "welcomed intruders" in the client's home; a positive outcome may be perceived by the client when he or she receives the care he or she wants and expects. The value the client assigns to that care is tied to mutually determining, with the caregiver, what the goals should be for the care provided. Being in the client's home, the caregiver is in a much better position to determine what is valued by the client, what is needed and wanted, and what resources are available to realistically achieve the outcomes desired than if that caregiver were in a hospital's sterile environment where the consumer is the guest. Although quality of care can be categorized in many ways, the clustering of attributes of quality is quite distinct from one consumer group to another. There is much about the determinants of performance that we do not understand. However, to the extent that consumers are demanding quality of care information and professionals are attempting to provide the services clients need to become as independent as possible, we must continue to use and refine the mechanisms that have been established by the professional and accrediting organizations, as well as by the federal and state governments.

DESIGNING A QUALITY ASSURANCE PROGRAM

Historically, quality assurance (QA) programs have failed because they were not based on the premise that quality is a multifaceted concept, defined by recipients, providers, and payers according to their perceptions of the quality of the service or performance. For each group, the term *quality* assumes a different meaning, which is buried in the value they place on the care provided; perceptions are critical to the success of monitoring and evaluating client care and provider performance for the purpose of sustained resolution of identified problems.

Perceptions of Quality

Clients want "competent and compassionate" care (Meisenheimer, 1987; Spiegel & Backhaut, 1980). They expect and value nurses who "take time to establish a 'caring', interpersonal relationship with them, . . . are accountable to them, and exhibit competence in assessing and managing their case, . . . while providing them with the care and information they need in a cost effective manner" (Meisenheimer, 1987, pp. 151–152). In defining quality, Donabedian (1982) has divided the management of an episode of illness into two domains (1) technical care, meaning the application of the science and technology of medicine, and (2) the accompanying interpersonal care, which manages the social and psychological interaction between client and practitioner. "Amenities," considered by Donabedian to be a third element of care, contribute to the management of the interpersonal relationship and are frequently noted in client/ practitioner satisfaction with the outcomes achieved. Since socially defined values and norms, including those dictated by the health profession, govern the interaction of individuals in both general and particular situations, it follows that the degree of quality in the management of the interpersonal relationship is measured by the extent of conformity to these values, norms, and expectations. While the degree to which the interpersonal relationship between clients and practitioners can influence the nature and success of the technical management of care is difficult to measure, attempts to do so are critical to the definition of quality. The confidence and trust that are assured through the development of the interpersonal relationship with the caregiver are essential to the client's perception and subsequent definition of quality.

As with clients, the interrelationship of Donabedian's two domains is reflected in nurses' and administrators' attempts to define quality. In taped interviews, Meisenheimer (1987) found that nurses expected their peers to be "competent in conducting a holistic assessment, . . . develop a positive interpersonal relationship with their clients, . . . be accountable for their practice, provide information to promote their client's independence, and manage the case to the client's satisfaction" (p. 152).

While administrators of home care agencies perceived the achievement of quality care similarly to nurses, cost efficiency and effectiveness are added dimensions (Meisenheimer, 1987). As health care providers facing sharp competition, administrators of home care agencies have responded to the reduced demand for inpatient care, the evolving revolution in how health services are being purchased, and the consumer interest in quality by marketing the clinical quality of a myriad of services. The quality benefit received for the price paid becomes a question of value. Although it is patently clear that quality and cost goals are unavoidably intertwined since services are often reimbursement-driven, rather than need-driven, the financial issues associated with home care will not be a major focus of this chapter.

Quality is in the mind of the beholder; reality is defined by each individual interacting in a given situation as s/he views it and acts on that perception. Individuals assess behaviors relative to arbitrary norms and standards and use such terms as *poor, fair,* and *good* to give meaning to those actions. Thus, the monitoring and evaluation of quality in home care must be examined from several perspectives—those of the client, the provider, and the agency. With heightened awareness of quality issues, these groups are defining and measuring quality, as well as making decisions on where to obtain health care and how to provide services based on both objective evidence and perceptions of quality (Hays, 1987). Recognizing the interrelatedness of these issues, an agency's mission statement or philosophy, which communicates to everyone what an agency will accomplish, provides the structure of the QA program. The purpose of the QA program is to monitor and evaluate the quality, appropriateness, and necessity of client care and provider performance for the purpose of improving client care.

Standards Governing Home Care

Being a highly regulated segment of the health care field, home health agencies have several professional, accrediting, state, and governmental sources for assistance with standards development. Agreed-on or expected levels of performance or conditions can be measured by the use of standards, a standard being any predetermined measure of extent, quantity, appropriateness, and/or quality. Standards reflect the values—the philosophy and goals—of an individual or organization and should provide the framework for designing a QA program. The inclusion of structure, process, and/or outcome standards as defined by Donabedian (1982) will ensure a comprehensive and effective approach to monitoring home care quality.

Professional Organizations

Professional organizations such as the American Nurses' Association (ANA) define standards as an "agreed upon level of excellence"; criteria are "statements which are measurable and which reflect the intent of the standard" (American Nurses' Association, 1986b). In 1986, the ANA published *Standards of Home Health Nursing Practice,* to be used in conjunction with *Standards of Community Health Nursing Practice.* Using a broadened approach to the development of standards to address structure, process, and outcome criteria, the 12 standards reflect two levels of practice: that of the generalist prepared at the baccalaureate level and that of the specialist prepared at the graduate level. (In the absence of the specialist, the generalist may assume aspects of the comprehensive role of the specialist.) The 12 standards, each with a rationale and with structure, process, and outcome criteria, address (1) organization of home health services, (2) theory, (3) data collection, (4) diagnosis, (5) planning, (6) intervention, (7) evaluation, (8) continuing of care including discharge planning and coordination of community services, (9) interdisciplinary collaboration, (10) professional development, (11) research, and (12) ethics (American Nurses' Association, 1986a).

The National League for Nursing (NLN) states that a standard "specifies the level of achievement a provider must abide by in order to become accredited" and that a criterion "describes the variable to be measured" (National League for Nursing, 1987, p. 39). A subsidiary of the NLN, the Community Health Accreditation Program (CHAP), was created in 1966 with the American Public Health Association and expanded in 1974. Its purpose is to assure quality in the long-term care setting, particularly in home- and community-based health care, through the active involvement of consumers. The accreditation process includes a self-study report, site visit, professional review panel, board of review, and inclusion in the listing of accredited agencies in NLN's publication *Nursing and Health Care*. CHAP's standards of excellence are moving toward outcome evaluation in addition to structure and process; they are not just minimum safety standards, but surpass the Omnibus Budget Reconciliation Act (OBRA) Medicare home care requirements (Mitchell, 1989).

In addition to the ANA and the NLN, the nursing profession is further governed by state licensure; the state nurse practice acts stipulate the basic minimum competency standards for the individual wishing to practice as a registered nurse. The issue of legal liability in the home health setting is of particular concern for nurses. While no court or jury has had to determine nursing accountability in caring for a client in his or her own home, the nursing care setting does relate to the applicable standard of care in that a nurse "is expected to act in a reasonable and prudent manner 'under the circumstances'" (Northrup, 1986, p. 252).

Standards of professional organizations usually focus on behaviors expected of the professional provider and consider the client's welfare. Serving as a model for professional practice, they request that quality go beyond the level of minimum regulatory standards.

Accrediting Agencies

In addition to the NLN's Community Health Accreditation Program (CHAP) noted previously, the Joint Commission on Accreditation of Healthcare Organizations provides a voluntary process by which a home care agency can be recognized as meeting predetermined standards and criteria (Joint Commission, 1988). Begun in early 1988, the Joint Commission's program includes high-tech infusion, durable medical equipment, homemaker services, home health aide services, and skilled professional care; observations of the client and staff in the home; client and staff interviews; and an audit of clinical records in every survey to assess the quality of administrative/management activities and clinical performance.

The National Home Caring Council, an accreditation program with 11 standards for homemaker and home health aide services, concentrates primarily on structure, staffing, service, and community. With an emphasis on training requirements for the homemaker and the home health aide, this accreditation program is consistent with state and federal requirements (Robinson, 1986).

Federal/State Standards

Since 1966, with the enactment of Medicare (Title 18 of the Social Security Act) and Medicaid (Title 19), the federal government has required a home health agency to meet "Conditions of Participation" in order to become a certified provider eligible to receive Medicare and Medicaid funds (Department of Health, Education, & Welfare, 1973; Webb, 1988). Focusing primarily on the provider's organizational structure, governance, and staffing patterns, the reviews by state surveyors serve to monitor compliance with state licensure, federal certification, and reimbursement guidelines.

The Omnibus Budget Reconciliation Act of 1986 (OBRA) required professional review organizations (PROs) to extend their reviews to home care. Effective April 1, 1989, PROs were required to review "Intervening Care"—that is, care that is delivered to a Medicare beneficiary by a home health agency between two prospective payment system (PPS) hospital admissions occurring within 31 calendar days. Generic quality screens, developed by the Health Care Financing Administration (HCFA), monitor whether the care provided met professionally recognized standards of care, services were timely and appropriate, and care was provided in an appropriate setting.

The minimum standards and criteria established by the federal and state licensing and certification agencies,have provided the basis for most QA programs. The private sector, including various fiscal intermediaries, is progressing toward Medicare guidelines as case managers are employed to monitor the quality of care being provided by home care agencies. Other organizations, as discussed by Schmele (1989) (i.e., the American Association of Retired Persons, National Council on Aging, National Consumer League, Hasting Center, and American Hospital Association, with their "patient bill of rights"), have delineated standards for safe, humane, and publicly accepted home health care. "The ideal standards implementation program will integrate agency values and mission, mandatory and reimbursement standards, and standards of the profession in such a way that the rights of clients to quality services will be clearly upheld'' (Schmele, 1989, p. 62).

Mission Statement/QA Program Purpose

A facility's mission statement communicates to the community what the members of a facility value and believe regarding client care—what they wish to accomplish. It may clarify respective roles for employees and clients. The QA program assists an agency in fulfilling its mission by monitoring its efforts toward providing an optimal level of performance and excellence.

The interrelatedness of the home health care agency's philosophy or mission statement may be stated thusly:

> The _____ Home Health Care Agency exists for the purpose of providing comprehensive, individually planned services to all clients in a changing environment supportive of excellence.

The QA program purpose may read as follows:

> The purpose of the quality assurance program is to assure the quality, appropriateness, and necessity of client care by systematically identifying and resolving known or potential problems.

Translating the mission statement into a QA program purpose should involve all members of the agency; enhancing acceptance and fostering ownership of the QA program will, to a greater degree, guarantee the implementation and success of the program. To be effective, the QA program should *never* be one person's responsibility; it should *never* respond *only* to the dictates of the state, the Joint Commission, or other accrediting and licensing/certifying agencies. It should reflect the expectations of these agencies in conjunction with the administration, employees, and consumers of services. A QA policy, as presented in Appendixes 8-A and 8-B, may serve to identify the program's purpose, objectives, responsible persons, and procedures and rationale for conducting various activities. Exhibit 8-1, a monitoring and evaluation calendar, establishes time frames for various activities. Risk management and utilization review activities should be included with quality assurance, as the three components comprise quality of care.

Monitoring and Evaluation

With the QA program's purpose, goals, and objectives clearly defined, the strategies that home care agencies adopt to assure the quality of professional

Exhibit 8-1 Monitoring and Evaluation Calendar

ACTIVITY	JAN	FEB	MAR	APR	MAY	JUNE	JULY	AUG	SEPT	OCT	NOV	DEC
Health Care Needs of Community	X											
Populations Served/Services/Visits Provided	X						X					
Staffing Policy/Procedure:												
#/Mix	X	X	X	X	X	X	X	X	X	X	X	X
Productivity	X			X			X			X	X	
Clinical Competence		X	X		X			X	X		X	
Generic Screens	X		X	X	X		X		X			
Clinical Study				X			X		X			
Care Plan Reviews	X	X	X	X	X	X	X	X	X	X	X	X
Nosocomial Infections	X	X	X	X	X	X	X	X	X	X	X	X
Medication Errors	X	X	X	X	X		X	X	X	X		
Incident Reports	X	X			X			X			X	
Documentation:												
Admission Assessments	X	X	X		X	X		X			X	X
Patient Education			X		X			X	X		X	
Client Outcomes Mutual Goals	X		X	X	X	X	X		X		X	X
Multidisciplinary Reviews	PT	OT	ST	PHAR	SS	C/S	PT	OT	ST	PHAR	SS	C/S
Client Satisfaction	X	X	X		X	X	X		X	X	X	
Physician Satisfaction						X	X			X		
Utilization Review	X		X			X		X			X	
Financial Management/Lost/Denied Charges	X		X		X	X	X	X			X	
Annual Review												

practices in home-delivered care must reflect the wide range of personnel and services (including contractual services) provided. The Joint Commission suggests choosing aspects of care that are high volume (occur frequently), high risk (may result in serious consequences if not performed properly), and/or problem-prone areas of concern. Some examples of indicators and thresholds (pre-established aggregate acceptable levels of performance) that trigger more intensive monitoring might include

- Patient education: Insulin-dependent diabetic patients
  Threshold for evaluation: 95 percent
- Infusion therapy
  Threshold for evaluation: 95 percent
- Wound care
  Threshold for evaluation: 90 percent
- Patient education in enterostomal care
  Threshold for evaluation: 90 percent
- Medication management
  Threshold for evaluation: 95 percent
- Infection control education in the care of the patient/client with AIDS
  Threshold for evaluation: 100 percent
- Medication management: Alzheimer's patients
  Threshold for evaluation: 100 percent
- Caregiver education in phototherapy treatment
  Threshold for evaluation: 100 percent
- Oxygen therapy
  Threshold for evaluation: 100 percent
- Continuity of care—Infusion therapy
  Threshold for evaluation: 80 percent
- Continuity of care—Multiple services
  Threshold for evaluation: 95 percent (Joint Commission, 1989)

QA STRATEGIES

In monitoring the chosen aspects of care, one must consider the consumer's demand for timely, appropriate care that preserves dignity and independence in addition to being scientifically correct; the caregiver's professional need for data on which to base practice decisions and articulate the domain of practice; and administration's need for input with regard to program evaluation, staff productivity, and resource allocation (Wilbert, 1985). Appropriate strategies might include the following.

Quality of Care Audit

A quality of care audit, as noted in a policy of the Visiting Nurse Association of Cleveland (Appendix 8-C, Exhibit 8-C-1), is done on a quarterly basis for the purpose of systematically evaluating the nursing care given to a randomly selected sample of discharged patients. Following the Guidelines for Completing Quality of Care Audit (Appendix 8-C, Exhibit 8-C-2), the assigned reviewer uses audit tools: (1) Knowledge Deficit Related to Diabetes Outcome Criteria (Appendix 8-C, Exhibits 8-C-3A and 8-C-4), and (2) Knowledge Deficit Related to Diabetes Nursing Process Criteria (Appendix 8-C, Exhibits 8-C-5A and 8-C-6B). The Quality of Nursing Care Audit Report (Appendix 8-C, Exhibit 8-C-7) was presented at the Patient Audit Committee (PAC) meeting. As noted in the policy, the director of QA/Utilization Review monitors the follow-up on corrective actions (Appendix 8-C, Exhibit 8-C-8), maintains a log of deficiencies and resolutions, and reports findings and recommendations to the chief executive officer and the Professional Advisory Board.

Quality of Specialty Nursing Care Audit

The Visiting Nurse Association of Cleveland provides examples of other quality of care evaluations as well. A Quality of Specialty Nursing Care Audit is done on a semiannual basis for the purpose of systematically evaluating the direct care given by intravenous therapists, enterostomal therapists, pediatric nurses, and geripsychiatric services. A sample of patients is randomly selected (Appendix 8-C, Exhibit 8-C-9), and the Procedure for Quality Assurance Peer Review Audit (Appendix 8-C, Exhibit 8-C-10) is followed. The aspect of care "Intravenous Therapy Services" is monitored using an audit tool (see Appendix 8-D and 8-E) that identifies the IV criteria and accepted threshold levels. The IV Quality of Care Audit Report (Exhibit 8-2) presented at the PAC meeting describes the purpose of the peer review, sample selection, findings, and recommendations. The Quality Assurance Peer Review Audit Follow-Up Action form (Exhibit 8-3) is confidential, not part of the patient's record, and should be used in a constructive manner for the purpose of improving professional practice.

Monitoring of Nursing Skills and Performance

Recipients of in-home services have been portrayed by the news media and legislative reports as frail, dependent clients, hidden away from public view.

Exhibit 8-2 IV Quality of Care Audit Report (For presentation at PAC Meeting on 7/20/89)

2ND QUARTER 1989	TOTAL AGENCY	# OF RECORDS REVIEWED: 10

SCOPE OF SERVICE: Intravenous Therapy Service

SEX:	Female	8	AGE:	Under 1 yr.	0
	Male	2		1–11	0
STATUS:				12–19	0
				20–34	0
	Active	3		35–49	2
	Discharged	7		50–64	2
				65–79	5
				80 and over	1

PURPOSE OF REVIEW:

Conduct peer review for monitoring and evaluating quality of intravenous therapy services given to a random sample of active and discharged patients.

SAMPLE SELECTION:

15% of the total number (65) of patients visited by IV therapists during March 1989 were randomly selected for a record audit. This sample is representative of all Centres.

REVIEWERS ASSIGNED:

The records were reviewed and data collection instruments for required key indicators or measurable criteria were completed by assigned IV therapists.

FINDINGS:

Criteria	Actual Performance	Threshold
Admission Screening	100%	100%
Physician Orders	100%	98%
Home Care Management	96%	99%
Safety	67%	100%
Infection Control	94%	100%
Complications	96%	100%
Emergency Measures	89%	100%
Response Time	N/A	92%
Overall Average	**92%**	**99%**

Of the 10 records reviewed 3 were active cases and 8 were female. 6 of the patients were 65 years of age and older and the median age was between 65 and 79 years of age.

2 of the 7 criteria evaluated were 100% met. The response time criterion was not evaluated during this audit as procedures for measuring this criterion have not been fully implemented. The safety criterion was unmet as 2 of 3 records did not show documentation regarding instruction on the use of rubbershod hemostats and 3 of 9 records indicated safe disposal of

continues

Exhibit 8-2 continued

needles. Infection control criteria were unmet as 2 of 10 records showed no documentation regarding handwashing and 1 of 2 records showed appropriate skin preparation with povodine prior to cannula insertion of a peripheral catheter site. Also, 2 of 4 records showed presence or absence of sutures and 2 of 3 cases indicated that patency of the central venous access was checked every visit. Complications criterion was unmet as only 2 of 3 cases showed documentation of ready availability of rubbershod hemostats when appropriate. Emergency measures criterion was unmet as only 4 of 6 records showed 24 hr. availability of supply company and pharmacist.

2 of the cases reviewed involved IV therapy services because of a difficult venipuncture; therefore, not all of the IV therapy audit tool criteria were appropriate for these cases and were rated not applicable.

Of the 8 cases requiring supervisory follow-up, 5 required action due to lack of documentation regarding safe disposal of needles and unclear understanding of the nurses' responsibility in arranging with the patient and/or family members how and where to discard needles safely. 2 of 6 cases requiring 24 hr. availability of supply company and pharmacist did not show evidence of compliance and required supervisory follow-up. Instances involving deficiencies related to broviac care and rubbershod hemostats and documentation of handwashing were followed up by the Directors of the Patient Care Centres with each IV therapist involved.

RECOMMENDATIONS:

1. That the Coordinator of IV Services and/or Director(s) of Patient Care Centres re-evaluate the IV therapy standardized Plans of Care and clinical documentation forms for adequacy of tool in documenting needle disposal practices and handwashing.
2. That the Coordinator of IV Services and/or Director(s) of Patient Care Centres review clinical practice policies and procedures related to safe disposal of needles.
3. That the Coordinator of IV Services and/or Director(s) of Patient Care Centres develop tools and procedures for tracking response time of the answering service and IV therapist.
4. That the Coordinator of IV Services develop an audit tool for phlebotomy cases to be used for the 4th Quarter IV Therapy Services Audit.

Source: Courtesy of the Visiting Nurse Association of Cleveland, Cleveland, OH.

Studies have shown that homemaker and home health aide services consistently account for 70 to 80 percent of all funds expended in the United States for home-delivered long-term care (Kemper, Applebaum, & Harrigan, 1987). For these reasons, but primarily because professionals are concerned about the quality of care provided to their clients, supervision of paraprofessional staff and monitoring of professional practice are critical. Exhibit 8-4 is an example of an audit tool that may be used by a supervisor to monitor and evaluate the care provided to clients by a home health aide (HHA) or a personal care aide (PCA). A performance evaluation tool (Exhibit 8-5) would be used by a supervisor and a professional nurse to jointly evaluate the nurse's skills and performance. Compliance with

Exhibit 8-3 Quality Assurance Peer Review Audit Follow-Up Action

PT   ST   IV   PEDS

OT   MSS   ET   GERIPSYCH (MH)
                    (circle one)

(This form is confidential and should not be part of the patient clinical record.)

STAFF ID# _____   REFERENCE DATE _____

PATIENT CASALUD# _____   CENTRE _____

A. Describe event, incident, or concern:

_____
Signature of Assigned
Reviewer/Title/Date

B. Specify recommendation/corrective action (include by whom and by when):

_____
Signature of Director of
QA/UR/Date

C. Specify response and follow-up action done (include by whom and by when):

_____
Signature of
Supervisor/Date

Source: Courtesy of the Visiting Nurse Association of Cleveland, Cleveland, OH.

Exhibit 8-4 Supervisory Visit: Home Health Aide/Personal Care Aide

HHA/PCA Name: _____   Date: _____

Initial Visit: _____ Repeat Visit: _____ Period of time being evaluated: _____

Client Name: _____   Visit/Frequency: _____ times weekly

Scope of Service: Home Health Aide/Personal Care Worker
Important Aspect of Care: Evaluation of HHA/PCW Skills & Performance
Quality of Care Indicators: Supervisor will visit HHA/PCW's clients 3 months following employment and at least every 6 months thereafter. HHA/PCW will perform tasks as demonstrated in orientation program.

PERFORMANCE CRITERIA	Excellent	Average	Poor	Comments
1. Personal Care:				
a. Bathing: bed; tub; shower; other				
b. Oral hygiene/Denture care				
c. Skin/Foot care				
d. Nail care				
e. Hair: brush; shampoo				
f. Shaving				
g. Dressing				
h. Catheter care				
i. Toileting				
j. Bed/Linen change				
2. Ambulation:				
a. Positioning				
b. Transfer: wheelchair; chair				
c. Walking: assistance; cane; walker; other				
d. Exercises: range of motion				
e. Restraints: safety belts, etc.				

continues

Exhibit 8-4 continued

PERFORMANCE CRITERIA	Excellent	Average	Poor	Comments
3. Nutrition:				
a. Diet preparation				
b. Feeding				
c. Intake/Output				
4. Additional Duties:				
a. Personal laundry				
b. Washing/Drying Dishes				
c. Dusting/Tidying client rm.				
d. Marketing				
e. Other (Specify)				
5. Safety/Infection Technique:				
a. Hand washing				
b. Disposal of contaminated supplies/equipment				
c. Uses equipment well				
d. Exercises personal safety				
e. Demonstrates good body mechanics				
f. Instructs client in proper usage of supplies/equipment				
6. Personal Characteristics of HHA/PCA:				
a. Greets client/family appropriately				
b. Explains purpose of visit				
c. Establishes rapport with client/family				

d. Able to give individual care to client satisfaction

e. Shows understanding of client's medical problem/needs

f. Personal appearance: appropriately attired; neat; clean

7. Additional Factors:

a. Follows nurse's care plan

b. Makes observations/assessments

c. Reports/Records unusual signs and symptoms of illness, changes in client's status to nurse

d. Documents care according to agency procedure

Additional Comments; Recommendations for Follow-up:

_____ _____
(HHA/PCA Signature)   (Date)

Comments: _____

_____ _____
(SUPERVISOR Signature)   (Date)

Exhibit 8-5 Performance Evaluation Tool

Scope of Service: Skilled Nursing Services

Important Aspect of Care: Evaluation of Monitoring of Nursing Skills and Performance

Quality of Care Indicators: All nurses receive a joint evaluation visit 3 months from the date of hire and at least annually thereafter.

PERFORMANCE EVALUATION CRITERIA	MET	UNMET	OTHER
1. *Preparation for Each Visit*			
A. Prescheduled visits with patients/families			
B. Obtained needed supplies			
C. Left completed schedule			
D. Scheduled visits in a systematic manner			
E. Researched diagnosis, medications, and treatments			
F. Comments _____			
2. *Home Visit*			
A. Greeted family/client appropriately			
B. Stated purpose of visit			
C. Carried out home visit in organized, logical manner			
D. Informed clients about each activity and received his/her consent			
E. Stated purpose for next home visit			
F. Remained flexible during visits adapting to the client's/family's needs			
G. Comments _____			
3. *Safety Factors*			
A. Hand washing done according to policy			
B. Proper bag technique employed			
C. Instructed patient in the proper use and maintenance of supplies and equipment			
D. Disposed of contaminated materials according to procedure			
E. Utilized office call-in procedure			
F. Exercised personal safety practice and awareness			
G. Comments _____			

continues

4. *Health Teaching, Guidance, and Counseling/Surveillance*
   A. Established/reviewed plan of care with client/family
   B. Utilized principles of adult learning
   C. Demonstrated care/treatments
   D. Comments _____

5. *Treatments and Procedures*
   A. Applied principles of asepsis and infection control
   B. Carried out medical orders
   C. Made observations/assessments in accordance with diagnosis and client need
   D. Planned interventions in accordance with diagnosis and client need
   E. Implemented interventions in accordance with diagnosis and client need
   F. Evaluated interventions in accordance with diagnosis and client need
   G. Comments _____

6. *Case Management*
   A. Utilized appropriate agency services
   B. Supervised HHA activities
   C. Reported pertinent findings to M.D.
   D. Utilized community resources
   E. Involved client/family in care
   F. Discharge planning evident
   G. Comments _____

7. *Documentation*
   A. Completed paperwork according to guidelines
   B. Documentation reflected changes in client's status
   C. Comments

Exhibit 8-5 continued

Comments and recommendations for follow-up:

PERFORMANCE EVALUATION CRITERIA: ☐ MET   ☐ UNMET

Supervisor Signature/Date _____

Employee Comments: _____

_____

_____

_____

_____

Employee Signature _____ Date

Source: Courtesy of the Visiting Nurse Association of Cleveland, Cleveland, OH.

performance evaluation criteria related to (1) the preparation for each visit; (2) the home visit itself; (3) safety factors; (4) health teaching, guidance, and counseling/ surveillance; (5) treatments and procedures; (6) case management; and (7) documentation are noted three months from the date of hire and at least annually thereafter. These data are critical to the enhancement of nursing practice.

Patient/Client Satisfaction Survey

While everyone is suggesting measurements of quality, the final judge of quality is the consumer—not a government report, an organization assessment, or a signed contract with a purchaser. The policy in the Patient/Client Satisfaction Survey (Appendix 8-F, Exhibit 8-F-1) and the Procedure for Completion of Patient Satisfaction Survey (Appendix 8-F, Exhibit 8-F-2) notes that the survey is given to each patient/or caregiver during the initial home visit and the completed survey is returned to the visiting nurse association at discharge. The stamped, self-addressed Patient Survey (Appendix 8-F, Exhibit 8-F-3) uses a Likert-type scale for respondents to rate the referral process, care provided by staff, and discharge process, and asks general questions about home care, as well as two open-ended questions asking for the client's comments. The Patient/Client Satisfaction Survey Report (Appendix 8-F, Exhibit 8-F-4) tabulates the responses to the various questions with greater elaboration under the ''Findings'' section.

Clients are indispensable sources of information in judging the quality of their care. They can verify, or fail to verify, the practitioner's reports or perceptions of care; they express satisfaction or dissatisfaction, passing judgment about many aspects of the process of care and its outcomes. If properly informed, clients can help regulate the quality of care by means of their choices. Client participation is necessary for the success of health care; it is clearly reflected by the outcomes of care.

CONCLUSION

Home health care is a complex process. The services actually received by a client are the end product of a complicated interplay of the application of relevant information and skills by the client, the individual practitioner, and teams of practitioners with policies and procedures of the health care organizations and agencies that finance and regulate health care. Each of the major participants in this scenario—client, practitioner, health care organization, purchaser, and regulator—views health care from a different perspective, and, therefore, they vary in their definitions of quality and how quality should be monitored and improved. Everyone does concur, however, that quality assurance is needed in health care.

Quality assurance programs must be practical, flexible, fair, and designed to achieve improvement in a priority fashion. They must receive organizational commitment and be designed to encompass the full spectrum of parameters of quality—from accessibility to satisfaction to conformance to contemporary scientific standards of care.

As we move into the twenty-first century, the access-cost-quality paradigm will continue to drive the health care system. Because the demand for home care services will only continue to grow, political and research reforms are required in the current system. In recognizing that health care is big business, and that home care is nursing care, nurses have an opportunity to manage their "product" and the available resources, balancing the value of business with the value of caring to build a solid foundation for success and survival. In recognizing that quality is something we are—exhibited in our behaviors—everyone will win, especially our clients.

REFERENCES

American Nurses' Association. (1986a). *Standards of home health nursing practice*. Kansas City, MO: Author.

American Nurses' Association. (1986b). *A plan for implementation of the standards of nursing practice*. Kansas City, MO: Author.

Applebaum, R., & Christianson, J. (1988). Using case management to monitor community-based long term care. *Quality Review Bulletin, 14*, 227–231.

Applebaum, R., & Wilson, N. (1988). Training needs for providing case management for the long term care client: Lessons from the national channeling demonstration. *Gerontologist, 28*(7), 172–176.

Department of Health, Education, and Welfare, Social Security Administration. (1973, July 16). Conditions of participation for home health agencies. *Federal Register, 38*(135).

Donabedian, A. (1982). *Explorations in quality assessment and monitoring* (Vol. 2). Ann Arbor, MI: Health Administration Press.

Elderly Health Services Letter. (1988, December). New Jersey: Elderly Health Services.

Hays, M. (1987). Consumers base quality perceptions on patient relations. *Modern Healthcare, 17*, 33.

Joint Commission on Accreditation of Healthcare Organizations. (1988). *Home care standards for accreditation*. Chicago: Author.

Joint Commission on Accreditation of Healthcare Organizations. (1989). *Quality assurance in home care: An introduction to a management process*. Chicago: Author.

Kemper, P., Applebaum, R., & Harrigan, M. (1987). *A systematic comparison of community care demonstrations*. Madison: University of Wisconsin, Institute for Research on Poverty.

Meisenheimer, C. (1987). Indices of quality in home health care: Perceptions of clients, nurses, and administrators. *Dissertation Abstracts International, 49*, 2594B.

Mitchell, M. (1989). The power of standards: The glory days of nursing yet to come? *Nursing and Health Care, 10*(6), 307–309.

Moore, F. (1988). *Homemaker and home health services: Policies and practices*. Owings Mills, MD: National Health Publishing.

National League for Nursing, Accreditation Division for Home Care and Community Health. (1987). *Accreditation criteria, standards, and substantiating evidences.* New York: Author.

Northrup, C. (1986). Home health care: Changing legal perspectives. *Nursing Outlook, 34*(5), 252.

Robinson, N. (1986). Standard setting and accreditation. *Caring, 5*(4), 34–39.

Schmele, J. (1989). Standards: The state of the art. In C. Meisenheimer (Ed.), *Quality assurance for home health care* (pp. 54–63). Gaithersburg, MD: Aspen Publishers.

Spiegel, A. (1987). *Home health care* (2nd ed.). Owings Mills, MD: National Health Publishing.

Spiegel, A., & Backhaut, B. (1980). *Curing and caring: A review of the factors affecting the quality and acceptability of health care.* Jamaica, NY: SP Medical & Scientific Books.

Stanhope, M. (1989). Home care: Past perspectives and implications for the present and future. In C. Meisenheimer (Ed.), *Quality assurance for home health care* (pp. 3–12). Gaithersburg, MD: Aspen Publishers.

U.S. Congress, House, Select Committee on Aging. (1985). *The fraudulent credentials hearing.* Washington, DC: U.S. Government Printing Office.

U.S. Congress, House, Select Committee on Aging. (1986). *The "black box" of home care quality.* Report prepared by the American Bar Association (Comm. Pub. 99-573). Washington, DC: U.S. Government Printing Office.

Webb, P. (1988). Adherence to conditions of participation. In M. Harris (Ed.), *Home health administration* (pp. 61–79). Owings Mills, MD: National Health Publishing.

Wilbert, C. (1985). Selecting topics/methodologies. In C. Meisenheimer (Ed.), *Quality assurance: A guide to effective programs* (p. 124). Gaithersburg, MD: Aspen Publishers.

Appendix 8-A

Quality Assurance Policy

Purpose: To systematically evaluate the quality of care rendered to individuals, families, and the community, in order to improve the quality of care provided, and to assure proper utilization of services.

Responsible Personnel: Nurses, Therapists, Social Workers, Members of the Professional Advisory Committee, Supervisors, Administrators, and Community Members

Objectives:
1. To assess and evaluate the quality and appropriateness of care.
2. To identify deviations from standards.
3. To address and resolve identified problems.
4. To recommend methods to improve care.

Policy: As we strive for excellence in the provision of care, the organization is committed to the development and implementation of a quality assurance program. The multifaceted program encompasses an ongoing evaluation of structural, process, and outcome criteria. To ensure quality-effective, cost-effective services (within available resources) to individuals, families, and the community, we subscribe to compliance with both internal and external standards. (Conditions of Participation, JCAHO, ANA, NAHC.)

Procedure:

Action	*Rationale*
A. *Quarterly Record Review*	
1. *Quarterly Periods*	1. Quarterly reports assess the
a. *1st Quarter*	services provided to
May—June—July	substantiate adherence to
(Quarterly report due by 3rd	agency policies, internal, and
Thursday in September)	external standards of services
b. *2nd Quarter*	for maintenance of optimal
Aug.—Sept.—Oct.	care, safety, and adequate
(Quarterly report due by 3rd	supportive services.
Thursday in December)	C.O.P. 484.52(b)

Source: Courtesy of the Visiting Nurse Association of Eastern Montgomery County; Department of Abington Memorial Hospital, Abington, PA.

172

Procedure: *Action*   *Rationale*

    c. *3rd Quarter*
      Nov.—Dec.—Jan.
      (Quarterly report due by 3rd
      Thursday in March)
    d. *4th Quarter*
      Feb.—March—April
      (Quarterly report due by 3rd
      Thursday in June)
    Annual report due 3rd Thursday in
    June.

2. The computer system generates a
   quarterly summary report which provides
   a numerical list of individuals serviced by
   all disciplines during the quarter. Based
   on these data, 10% of the records (7% if
   the caseload is greater than 500) to a
   maximum of 50 per discipline per quarter
   are chosen. If the number is less than 10
   cases per discipline for the quarter, all
   records for that discipline will be
   reviewed.

3. Records for review are selected randomly
   from the quality assurance review list, the
   visit register, and/or the active and
   discharged chart files.

4. Recording of individual record findings
   and recommendations on quality
   assurance assessment forms are
   implemented with 3 weeks notice as
   follows:
   a. Nursing and HHA: Nursing staff,
      supervisors, nurse volunteers.
   b. Physical therapy: Physical
      therapists—no one will review
      their own record.
   c. MSS: Review with neighboring home
      care agency.
   d. Speech Pathology: Review by
      speech contractor.
   e. Occupational Therapy: Alternate
      between contractors.

5. A summary of findings and
   recommendations are recorded in:
   a. Committee quarterly minutes and
      PAC minutes.
   b. Annual report to PAC at end of
      4th quarter as part of agency's
      program evaluation.

5. This summary complies with
   Medicare Conditions of
   Participation.

Procedure: *Action*   *Rationale*

6. A summary of findings is presented to staff members.

6. The staff uses the summary report to identify areas of strengths and weaknesses, then recommend and initiate action for the enhancement of care.

B. *Discharged Patient Questionnaires*
1. Each month, discharged patient questionnaires are mailed to 10% of the patients/families listed on the discharged patient computer list.

1. These questionnaires provide data to evaluate patient satisfaction with services provided.

2. The QA supervisor reviews each questionnaire. If a problem area is identified, it is addressed with the appropriate employee and supervisory staff, if indicated. Compliments to individuals are shared with individual and supervisory staff when indicated.

2. This review provides for follow up on patient responses.

3. The QA supervisor tallies the results of the survey and prepares a summary report for the executive director. These summaries may be utilized in the overall agency evaluation.

3. This summary is utilized in the overall program evaluation.

C. *Unsolicited Letters*
1. Unsolicited patient, family, community group letters are read and analyzed. Praise and/or problems are directed to and addressed with the appropriate persons by the QA supervisor. Comments that the writer shares about services and/or personnel are reviewed and taken into consideration to praise employees and/or address and correct cited problems.

1. The patient has the right to direct comments concerning quality of care to the organization.

D. *Annual Physician Questionnaires*
1. On an annual basis, questionnaires are mailed to physicians whose patients require a recertification of a plan of treatment during a 62-day cycle. Any necessary follow up is directed by the QA supervisor

1. These questionnaires encourage physician input as to their perception of the quality of services, since a physician who perceives the organization as providing quality care is more apt to refer his or her patients for services.

E. *Utilization Review*
1. Utilization is linked to the quality of services. Utilization of services is evaluated during the quarterly review

1. This review ensures proper utilization of all disciplines and services.

Procedure: *Action*   *Rationale*

process. Refer to Utilization Review
Policy, #3.15.

F. *Annual Program Evaluation*

 1. The Professional Advisory committee,   1. Annual evaluation is required
    administration, and staff are involved   by Medicare C.O.P. 484.52
    in the evaluation process as detailed in   to assess the extent to which
    the Annual Program Evaluation   the program services are
    Policy, #1.14. Within 90 days of the   appropriate, adequate,
    close of the fiscal year, representatives   effective, and efficient.
    from PAC meet to complete the
    necessary worksheets.
    A summary of the evaluation is
    presented to the PAC.

G. *Evaluation of Clinical Competence*

 1. Hiring practices are in accordance   1. To meet C.O.P. 484.4 from
    with C.O.P. 484.4.   a structural perspective.
                                                  Clinical competence and
                                                  education are necessary to
                                                  provide quality care.

 2. Copies of licenses, when applicable,   2. To meet C.O.P. 484.4 from
    are on file. Certification, where   a structural perspective.
    applicable (i.e., ANA certification for   Clinical competence and
    community health nurse), is   education are necessary to
    encouraged.   provide quality care.

 3. Each employee/volunteer is oriented   3. To meet C.O.P. 484.4 from
    to his or her roles and responsibilities.   a structural perspective.
                                                  Clinical competence and
                                                  education are necessary to
                                                  provide quality care.

 4. Continuing education is linked to the   4. To meet C.O.P. 484.4 from
    quality assurance program to ensure   a structural perspective.
    that training is commensurate with   Clinical competence and
    quality care needs.   education are necessary to
                                                  provide quality care.

 5. Licenses are verified on all physicians   5. To meet C.O.P. 484.4 from
    ordering home care services.   a structural perspective.
                                                  Clinical competence and
                                                  education are necessary to
                                                  provide quality care.

 6. Physician management of home care   6. This evaluation will be done
    patients will be evaluated on a   by a subcommittee of PAC.
    periodic basis and for selected cases.

H. *Monitor and Review of Patient Outcome*

 1. Services are goal oriented. Outcomes   1. These steps evaluate goal
    are addressed through the use of a   attainment and ensure that
    patient classification system and   quality care was rendered.
    nursing diagnoses. Staff must quantify
    goal attainment. Financial and clinical

Procedure: *Action*   *Rationale*

         goal attainment data are available on a
         monthly basis through the
         Management Information System
         printouts. Data are analyzed on a
         periodic basis. Results are shared with
         appropriate staff members.

I. *Incident Reports*

   1. Any staff involved in an incident   1. Trends in reportable
      completes an incident report and   incidents are a quality
      submits it to the Director of   assurance/risk management
      Professional Services. Trends   concern and should be
      identified are given to the QA   studied and acted upon.
      supervisor for further study and follow
      up.

J. *Assessment of Important Aspects of Care*

   1. Refer to Quality Assurance plan for   1. Ongoing and systematic
      important aspects of care.   assessment of important
                             aspects of care and quality
                             indicators is conducted to
                             identify and resolve problems
                             in structure, process, or
                             outcome.

COP 484.16; 484.52

JCAHO   Origin date: 11/87
          Revised date: 9/88; 8/89
          Approved by: Administration/Board/PAC/AMH QA Committee
          Originator: Administration
          Distribution: Administration/Staff/Contractors/PAC/Volunteers

Appendix 8-B

Annual Program Evaluation Policy

DEFINITION OF PROGRAM EVALUATION:

Program evaluation is the systematic collection and analysis of information necessary to assess agency effectiveness, quality, and efficiency relative to accepted performance measures and standards, and to guide agency planning for the provision of health care to those it serves.

GOALS OF AGENCY EVALUATION

A. To assess and improve the quality of agency programs and services.
B. To assure the relevance of all agency programs and services to community needs.
C. To accomplish and maintain overall agency accountability for programs and services.
D. To document and facilitate the prudent utilization of resources in the operation of agency programs and services.
E. To achieve and maintain the relevance of agency programs and services to the agency mission.

UNIFORM PROGRAM EVALUATION CRITERIA

A. *Scope*
    1. The annual program evaluation will include an assessment of all programs and services offered by the agency both directly (i.e., by employed staff) and through contract in a twelve-month period comprising the program year.
    2. The annual program evaluation shall address the following elements of the agency: (I) administration and organization; (II) staffing; (III) programs and services; and (IV) the status of future agency plans bearing on service delivery and/or quality.
    3. The annual program evaluation will provide for an assessment of the adequacy, appropriateness, effectiveness, efficiency, and competency of health care delivery to agency patients and other service beneficiaries.
B. *Responsibility*
    1. The procedure for the Annual Evaluation specifies which personnel, group, or committees participate in the process.

Source: Courtesy of the Visiting Nurse Association of Eastern Montgomery County, Abington, PA.

2. The Board of Directors, Professional Advisory Committee, administration, and staff are involved in the evaluation process.

C. *Required Annual Reviews*

1. The annual program evaluation will document and appraise the conformance of agency program operations with policies established by the Board of Directors and approved by the Professional Advisory Committee.

2. The annual program evaluation will include an assessment of patient care activities through a review of clinical records performed on an appropriate sample basis in relation to the Clinical Record Audit and Utilization Review functions of the agency.

3. The annual program evaluation will provide a basis for assessing overall agency program operations in terms of economy and efficiency in relation to cost containment and cost effectiveness.

D. *Format and Organization*

1. The annual program evaluation will be presented in a written format indicating those involved, general methods and procedures, specific findings or results, and any comments regarding corrective action or recommendations for further improvement.

2. The annual program evaluation report will also address the disposition of any specific findings or recommendations presented in previous agency evaluation reports.

E. *External Feedback*

1. The annual program evaluation process will involve a formal method of determining patient satisfaction with the services provided by the agency. Comments should be gathered directly from the patients or their representatives.

2. The annual program evaluation process will include a means of collecting information on agency program performance from the physicians of patients served by the agency.

3. The annual program evaluation process will provide for the collection of information from sources such as hospitals, other health care providers, social agencies, and similar entities concerning agency performance in accepting and follow-up with referrals for service when appropriate.

F. *Integration with Agency Accreditation*

The documentation requirements for initial and ongoing voluntary accreditation under the National League for Nursing/Community Health Accreditation Program are recognized as fully consistent with above-stated criteria. The comprehensive self-study report that is prepared for interim and renewal of accreditation will be utilized for program evaluation purposes for the years covered.

Appendix 8-C

Examples of Studies

Subject: QUALITY OF CARE AUDIT	Policy #
Authorizing Signature: Title:	Supersedes Policy # Dated 10/1/88
Concurrence:	Effective Date: 5/2/89

CHIEF EXECUTIVE OFFICER:

A Quality of Care Audit is done on a quarterly basis for the purpose of systematically evaluating the nursing care given to a randomly selected sample of discharged patients.

The Director of QA/UR monitors the follow-up on corrective actions, maintains a log of deficiencies and resolutions, and reports findings and recommendations to the Chief Executive Officer and the Professional Advisory Committee.

Source: Courtesy of the Visiting Nurse Association of Cleveland, Cleveland, OH.

Exhibit 8-C-2 Guidelines for Completing Quality of Care Audit Follow-Up Action Form

This form is confidential and should not be part of the patient's clinical record. Also, no patient or staff should be identified except by number.

When any unmet outcome or nursing process criteria is identified by the assigned reviewer, the reviewer completes this form for the Director of Quality Assurance. The identifying data are taken from the audit tools and the Reference Date is a combination of the Start of Care (SOC) and Discharge (DC) dates. For example, 01/02/88—02/15/88.

Event, incident, or concern:

The assigned reviewer briefly describes why the criterion was considered to be unmet. Be as specific as possible so that the Quality of Care Audit Committee has pertinent, critical information for recommendation of corrective action. The assigned reviewer then signs and dates (including Title).

Recommendations/corrective action:

This section is completed by the Director of Quality Assurance. Recommendation for corrective action is stated including who should follow up and by when and is signed and dated (including Title).

Response and follow-up action done:

This section is completed by the person assigned to follow up on the deficiency and corrective action and is signed and dated (including Title).

Source: Courtesy of the Visiting Nurse Association of Cleveland, Cleveland, OH.

Exhibit 8-C-3 Knowledge Deficit Related to Diabetes Outcome Criteria

Casalud# _____ Team _____ ICD-9 _____ Referral Source _____
(vo)
Sex _____ Age _____ Adm. Date _____ DC Date _____ DC Code _____ DOS _____

Cond. on DC _____ Date of Last Visit _____ Staff #_____

MD notified of DC?   Y   N   Date MD notified _____
(circle one)
Notification charted on narrative?   Y   N   (circle one)

Patient/caregiver demonstrates:

	MET	UNMET	OTHER
Knowledge of disease			
Correct glucose monitoring			
Recognition s/sx hypo-hyperglycemia			
Correct procedure for insulin adm.			
Describe meds			
Diet/meal preparation			
Prevention/control of complications			
Acceptable blood sugar			
Adaptive coping mechanisms			
Plan for medical follow-up			
When to seek medical advice or follow-up			
Knowledge re community resources			

OUTCOME CRITERIA: ☐ MET   ☐ UNMET

_____
Reviewer's Signature   Date
and Title

Source: Courtesy of the Visiting Nurse Association of Cleveland, Cleveland, OH.

Exhibit 8-C-4 Thresholds for Knowledge Deficit Related to Diabetes Outcome Criteria

Patient/caregiver demonstrates:

	THRESHOLD
Knowledge of disease	85%
Correct glucose monitoring	100%
Recognition s/sx hypo-hyperglycemia	85%
Correct procedure for insulin adm.	100%
Describe meds	85%
Diet/meal preparation	85%
Prevention/control of complications	80%
Acceptable blood sugar	85%
Adaptive coping mechanisms	85%
Plan for medical follow-up	85%
When to seek medical advice or follow-up	85%
Knowledge re community resources	85%
Average	87%

Source: Courtesy of the Visiting Nurse Association of Cleveland, Cleveland, OH.

Exhibit 8-C-5 Knowledge Deficit Related to Diabetes Nursing Process Criteria

Nurse will assess/instruct in the following:	MET	UNMET	OTHER
Vital signs			
Glucose level/glucose monitoring			
Weight			
Signs & symptoms of hypo/hyperglycemia			
Prescribed diet			
Preparation and administration of insulin			
Disease process			
Complications			
Circulatory changes			
Skin integrity			
Foot and skin care			
Medication regimen			
Coping mechanisms			
Reduction of risk factors			
Regular medical follow-up			
When to seek medical advice/emergency care			
Obtain lab work as ordered			
Refer to available resources			

PROCESS CRITERIA: ☐ MET   ☐ UNMET

Reviewer's Signature   Date
and Title

Source: Courtesy of the Visiting Nurse Association of Cleveland, Cleveland, OH.

Exhibit 8-C-6 Thresholds for Knowledge Deficit Related to Diabetes Nursing Process Criteria

	THRESHOLD
Nurse will assess/instruct in:	
Vital signs	100%
Glucose level/glucose monitoring	100%
Weight	100%
Signs & symptoms of hypo/hyperglycemia	100%
Prescribed diet	100%
Preparation and administration of insulin	100%
Disease process	100%
Complications	85%
Circulatory changes	85%
Skin integrity	85%
Foot and skin care	85%
Medication regimen	100%
Coping mechanisms	85%
Reduction of risk factors	85%
Regular medical follow-up	85%
When to seek medical advice/emergency care	100%
Obtain lab work as ordered	100%
Refer to available resources	85%
Average	93%

Source: Courtesy of the Visiting Nurse Association of Cleveland, Cleveland, OH.

Exhibit 8-C-7 Quality of Nursing Care Audit Report (For presentation at PAC Meeting on 7/20/89)

2ND QUARTER 1989			**# of Discharged Records Reviewed**: 27		
SCOPE OF SERVICE: Skilled Nursing					

Sex: Female	18	**AGE:** Under 1 yr.	0
Male	9	1–11	1
		12–19	0
Days of Stay (DOS):		20–34	1
1–30 days	16	35–49	2
31–60	5	50–64	4
61–90	2	65–79	13
91–120	1	80 and over	6
121–150	1		
Over 150 days	2		

Referral Source:

Hosp. Inpatient	18	Physician	1	Comm. Ag.	0
Outpatient	5	SNF/NH	1	Other	0
Contract Hosp.	14	Patient/Family	2		

Purpose of Review:

Conduct peer review for monitoring and evaluating quality of nursing care given to a sample of patients diagnosed with diabetes mellitus.

Sample Selection:

100% of April 1989 discharged patients with a primary medical diagnosis of diabetes mellitus, with or without complications, and insulin- and noninsulin-dependent were selected for a process and outcome peer review. The sample is also representative of patients referred by contract institutions. This group of patients was selected on the basis of high risk, high volume population and an evaluation of quality of care prior to the scheduled diabetes workshop in the fall of 1989. This is a higher priority than the nursing diagnoses identified resulting from the 2nd quarter quality of care evaluation audit.

Reviewers Assigned:

The records were reviewed and data collection instruments for required key indicators were completed by assigned registered nurses.

Findings:

18 of the 27 reviewed discharged patients were female and 19 were 65 years of age or older. The median age range was 65 to 79 years of age. 16 patients were under care for 30 days or less and 4 patients were under care for longer than 90 days.

19 were referred to the VNA following hospital or extended care/nursing home stays. Two patients were referred by family members. 14 of the patients were referred by contract institutions.

continues

Exhibit 8-C-7 continued

Knowledge Deficit Related to Diabetes Criteria	Actual Performance	Threshold (Level of Acceptance)
HEIGHTS CENTRE		
1. Process	72%	93%
2. Outcome	75%	87%

Knowledge Deficit Related to Diabetes Criteria	Actual Performance	Threshold (Level of Acceptance)
OHIO CITY CENTRE		
1. Process	96%	93%
2. Outcome	97%	87%

Knowledge Deficit Related to Diabetes Criteria	Actual Performance	Threshold (Level of Acceptance)
TOTAL AGENCY		
1. Process	87%	93%
2. Outcome	85%	87%

12 of 18 process criteria and 7 of 12 outcome criteria were 100% met. Because of the vast differences in actual performances between the two Centres, there is a question of a problem in the review process itself rather than a question of the quality of clinical practice of each Centre staff.

Recommendations:

1. That the Clinical Services Committee assess and evaluate the review process and rating decisions.
2. That reviewers be reinstructed regarding the quality of care audit process.
3. That the same nursing diagnosis quality of care audit be repeated next quarter.

Source: Courtesy of the Visiting Nurse Association of Cleveland, Cleveland, OH.

Exhibit 8-C-8 Quality of Care Audit Follow-Up Action

(This form is confidential and should not be part of the patient clinical record.)

STAFF ID# _____   REFERENCE DATE _____

PATIENT CASALUD# _____ CENTRE _____ ICD9 CODE _____

A. Describe event, incident, or concern:

                                    _____
                                    Signature of Assigned
                                    Reviewer/Title/Date

B. Specify recommendation/corrective action (include by whom and by when):

                                    _____
                                    Signature of Director of
                                    QA/UR/Date

C. Specify response and follow-up action done (include by whom and by when):

                                    _____
                                    Signature of
                                    Supervisor/Date

Source: Courtesy of the Visiting Nurse Association of Cleveland, Cleveland, OH.

Exhibit 8-C-9 Visiting Nurse Association of Cleveland Policy Manual: Quality of Specialty
Nursing Care Audit

SUBJECT: Quality of Specialty Nursing Care Audit	Policy #
Authorizing Signature: Title:	Supersedes Policy #
Concurrence:	Effective Date: 5/2/89

| Chief Executive Officer: | |

A Quality of Specialty Nursing Care Audit is done on a semiannual basis for the purpose of systematically evaluating the direct care given by intravenous therapists, enterostomal therapists, pediatric nurses, and geripsychiatric services to a randomly selected sample of patients.

The Director of QA/UR monitors the follow-up on corrective actions, maintains a log of deficiencies and resolutions, and reports findings and recommendations to the Chief Executive Officer and the Professional Advisory Committee.

Source: Courtesy of the Visiting Nurse Association of Cleveland, Cleveland, OH.

Exhibit 8-C-10 Procedure for Quality Assurance Peer Review Audit

1. The Director of QA/UR selects a random sample of 10% of the patients visited by a specified allied health or specialty nursing services staff during a given month.
2. The sample is representative of the distribution of patients by centre and the patients selected may be active or discharged.
3. The Director of Patient Centre(s) is notified by memo of what records need to be pulled for the reviewer.
4. The Director of Allied Health Services or Coordinator for Specialty Nursing Care is responsible for the peer review of the clinical record.
5. The completed audit tool is left attached to the record and the Director of Allied Health Services or Coordinator notifies the Director of QA/UR when the review is complete.
6. The Director of QA/UR reviews the completed tool and makes recommendations on the Quality Assurance Peer Review Audit Follow-Up Action form.
7. The Director of QA/UR monitors the follow-up on corrective actions, maintains a log of deficiencies and resolutions, and reports findings and recommendations to the Chief Executive Officer and the Professional Advisory Committee.

Source: Courtesy of the Visiting Nurse Association of Cleveland, Cleveland, OH.

Appendix 8-D

Aspects of Care for Intravenous Therapy Services

Scope of Service: Nursing Services

Important Aspect of Care: Intravenous Therapy Services

Quality of Care Indicators: All patients who receive intravenous therapy must meet the IV therapy criteria.

CENTRE _____ CASALUD# _____ AGE _____ SEX _____

IV THERAPY CRITERIA:	MET	UNMET	OTHER
1. *Admission Screening*			
A. Received medications & blood components in a controlled environment 24 hrs. prior to at home reception			
2. *Physician Orders*			
A. All IV orders are verbal/signed by physician responsible for infusion therapy			
B. Orders include			
1. Type of therapy			
2. Name & dosage and/or amount of medications/fluids			
3. How often it is to be given and for how long			
4. Any emergency care for treatment of extravasation			
5. Any specific lab work			

3. *Home Care Management*
   A. Patient or caregiver verbalizes basic knowledge of infusion controller, drug-related complications, and how to obtain emergency service.
   B. Supplies & equipment were ordered as needed
   C. Environment adapted for storage of equipment & medication
   D. Infusion controllers functioned properly
   E. Medical follow-up
   F. Patient or CG taught how to recognize the following:
      1. S/sx of infiltration
      2. How & when to discontinue infusion or cannula
      3. S/sx of infection or phlebitis
      4. Use of rubbershod hemostats (for broviac only)
   G. Provision of emotional support
   H. Obtain lab work as ordered by physician

4. *Safety*
   A. Disposable needle container available in the home
   B. Proper storage of fluids and/or medications
   C. For transfusion therapy only
      1. Monitor vital signs
         a. Prior to administration
         b. Every 15 minutes ×2
         c. Every 30 minutes during transfusion
         d. Upon completion of transfusion
      2. Visited later in week to assess for signs of delayed transfusion reaction: e.g., infection, fever

5. *Infection Control*
   A. Hand washing
   B. Monitor vital signs and physical status of patient every visit (VS's exception for BID or TID visit; then QD)
   C. Change tubing QD for TPN & all medications
   D. Change tubing q 48 hrs. for hydration only

Source: Courtesy of the Visiting Nurse Association of Cleveland, Cleveland, OH.

continues

	MET	UNMET	OTHER

IV THERAPY CRITERIA:

E. Peripheral Catheter Site
1. Skin prepped with povodine prior to cannula insertion
2. Occlusive transparent dressing changed q 48–72 hrs.
3. Condition of site observed each visit
4. Antecubital fossa not a site recommended
5. Phlebitis prevention
   a. Catheter changed every 72 hrs. or MD order stating change to be less frequently
   b. Tubing changed q 24–48 hrs.
   c. Patency checked q visit
   d. Patient recognizes and reports symptoms of infiltration

F. Central Venous Access (Broviac/Hickman)
1. Occlusive transparent dressing changed M–W–F (3 times/week) and as needed
2. Observe condition of exit site each visit
3. Patient recognizes & reports s/sx of infection
4. Change male adapters q week
5. Presence or absence of sutures
6. Patency checked every visit

G. Implanted Access Device
1. Monitor for redness, edema, swelling, tissue breakdown
2. Occlusive transparent dressing change q week or as needed
3. Frequency of male adaptor plug and leur lock change
4. Huber needle changed q week & prn
5. Patency checked q visit

6. Complications

A. Patient to recognize report s/sx of infiltration

B. Patency checked each visit
1. Flush with normal saline, 1–2cc, Saline Antibiotic Saline Heparin (SASH)
2. At end of infusion, flush with normal saline, 1–2cc, followed by 100u/ml of Heparin flush 2–3cc (SASH method)

For Mediport:
1. Flush with normal saline prior to each infusion
2. Per order flush with 3–5cc./100u/1ml heparin post infusion and/or q month whichever comes 1st.

C. Air embolism (Broviac)
   1. Patient must have rubbershod hemostats readily available
   2. Patient should be able to verbalize and demonstrate proper clamping of catheter

D. Drug reaction
   1. Observe for s/sx q visit and report any adverse reaction to the physician

7. *Emergency Measures*
   A. Visiting nurse available 24 hrs.
   B. Local emergency #911
   C. Supply company & pharmacist available 24 hrs.

8. *Response Time**
   A. Answering service log of IV calls
      1. Patient's name
      2. Date
      3. Time of call
      4. Time nurse paged
      5. Time nurse responded
   B. IV coordinator's log
      1. Patient's name
      2. Date
      3. Time received call from answering service
      4. Time nurse called patient

*All on-call response time will be less than 20 minutes (evenings, nights, weekends, and holidays).

Comments and recommendations for follow-up:

☐ MET   ☐ UNMET

IV CRITERIA:

_____   Date
Signature of Reviewer/Title

Appendix 8-E

Intravenous Therapy Criteria

IV THERAPY CRITERIA:	THRESHOLD
1. *Admission Screening*	100%
A. Received medications & blood components in a controlled environment prior to at home reception	100%
2. *Physician Orders*	100%
A. IV orders are signed by physician responsible for infusion therapy	100%
B. Orders include	
1. Type of therapy	100%
2. Name & dosage and/or amount of medication/fluids	100%
3. How often it is to be given and for how long	100%
4. Any emergency care for treatment of extravasation	100%
5. Any specific lab work	100%
3. *Home Care Management*	99%
A. Patient or caregiver verbalizes basic knowledge of infusion controller drug, related complications, and how to obtain emergency service.	100%
B. Supplies & equipment were ordered as needed	100%
C. Environment adapted for storage of equipment & medication	100%
D. Infusion controllers functioned properly	100%
E. Medical follow-up	100%
F. Patient taught how to recognize the following:	
1. S/sx of infiltration	100%
2. How & when to discontinue infusion or cannula	100%
3. S/sx of infection or phlebitis	100%
4. Use of rubbershod hemostats (for broviac only)	100%
G. Provision of emotional support	90%
H. Obtain lab work as ordered by physician	100%
4. *Safety*	100%
A. Disposable needle container available in the home	100%
B. Proper storage of fluids and/or medications	100%

Source: Courtesy of the Visiting Nurse Association of Cleveland, Cleveland, OH.

IV THERAPY CRITERIA:	THRESHOLD

C. For transfusion therapy only:

  1. Monitor vital signs

a. Prior to administration	100%
b. Every 15 minutes × 2	100%
c. Every 30 minutes during transfusion	100%
d. Upon completion of transfusion	100%
2. Visited later in week to assess for signs of delayed transfusion reaction:	100%
e.g., infection, fever	
5. *Infection Control*	100%
A. Hand washing	100%
B. Monitor vital signs and physical status of patient every visit (VS's exception	100%
for BID or TID visit; then QD)	
C. Change tubing QD for TPN & all medications	100%
D. Change tubing q 48 hrs. for hydration only	100%
E. **Peripheral Catheter Site**	
1. Skin prepped with povodine prior to cannula insertion	100%
2. Occlusive transparent dressing changed q 48–72 hrs.	100%
3. Condition of site observed each visit	100%
4. Antecubital fossa not a site recommended	100%
5. Phlebitis prevention	
a. Catheter changed every 72 hrs. or MD order stating change to be less	100%
frequently	
b. Tubing changed q 24–48 hrs.	100%
c. Patency checked q visit	100%
d. Patient recognizes and reports symptoms of infiltration	100%
F. **Central Venous Access (Broviac/Hickman)**	
1. Occlusive transparent dressing M–W–F (3 times a week) and as needed	100%
2. Observe condition of exit site each visit	100%
3. Patient recognizes & reports s/sx of infection	100%
4. Change male adapters once a week	100%
5. Presence or absence of sutures	100%
6. Patency checked every visit	100%
G. **Implanted Access Device**	
1. Monitor for redness, edema, swelling, tissue breakdown	100%
2. Occlusive transparent dressing change q week or as needed	100%
3. Frequency of male adapter plug & leur lock change	100%
4. Huber needle changed q week & prn	100%
5. Patency checked q visit	100%
6. *Complications*	100%
A. Patient to recognize and report s/sx of infiltration	100%
B. Patency checked each visit:	
1. Flush with normal saline, 1–2cc, Saline Antibiotic Saline Heparin	100%
(SASH)	
2. At end of infusion, flush with saline, 1–2cc, followed by 100u/ml of	100%
Heparin flush, 2–3cc (SASH method)	
For Mediport:	
1. Flush with normal saline prior to each infusion	100%
2. Per order flush with 3–5cc/100u/ml heparin post infusion and/or q month	100%
whichever comes 1st.	

IV THERAPY CRITERIA: **THRESHOLD**

  C. Air embolism (Broviac)
    1. Patient must have rubbershod hemostats readily available   100%
    2. Patient should be able to verbalize and demonstrate proper clamping of 100%
       catheter
  D. Drug Reaction
    1. Observe for s/sx q visit and report any adverse reaction to the physician 100%
7. *Emergency Measures*   100%
  A. Visiting nurse available 24 hrs.   100%
  B. Local emergency #911   100%
  C. Supply company & pharmacist available 24 hrs.   100%
8. *Response Time**   92%
  A. Answering service log of IV calls: 90%
    1. Patient's name   90%
    2. Date   90%
    3. Time of call   90%
    4. Time nurse paged   90%
    5. Time nurse responded   90%
  B. IV coordinator's log of IV calls:
    1. Patient's name   95%
    2. Date   95%
    3. Time received call from answering service   95%
    4. Time nurse called patient   95%

*All on-call response time will be less than 20 minutes (evenings, nights, weekends, and holidays).

Source: Courtesy of the Visiting Nurse Association of Cleveland, Cleveland, OH.

Appendix 8-F

Examples of Patient/Client Satisfaction Surveys

Exhibit 8-F-1 The Visiting Nurse Association Policy Manual: Patient/Client Satisfaction Survey

Subject: Patient/Client Satisfaction Survey	**Policy #**
Authorizing Signature: **Title:**	**Supersedes** **Policy #**
Concurrence:	**Effective Date:**
Chief Executive Officer:	

For the purpose of promoting quality of care, a Patient Satisfaction Survey is given to each patient/or caregiver during the initial home visit for completion and return to the Visiting Nurse Association at discharge.

The Director of Quality Assurance/Utilization Review reviews the returned surveys, makes recommendations, tabulates the data, monitors the follow-up, maintains a log of deficiencies and corrective actions, writes and submits reports.

Source: Courtesy of the Visiting Nurse Association of Cleveland, Cleveland, OH.

Exhibit 8-F-2 Procedure for Completion of Patient Satisfaction Survey Quality Assurance Activity

1. Patient Satisfaction Survey form is placed in each admission packet and given to the patient/ client or caregiver during the initial home visit.
2. Patient/client or caregiver is given an explanation of the purpose and confidentiality of the survey and is requested to complete the survey as frankly as desired and to return it when the patient is discharged.
3. The Case manager reminds the family to return the form when the last visit is made.
4. The Director of Quality Assurance/Utilization Review reviews the returned surveys, makes recommendations when necessary, tabulates the data, monitors the follow-up, and maintains a log of deficiencies and corrective actions.
5. On a regular basis the Chief Executive Officer is given feedback.
6. Each Quarter, the Director of Quality Assurance/Utilization Review submits a report of findings and recommendations.
7. The Director and Supervisors will have access to the forms on a regular basis in addition to reports.
8. When a deficiency or quality of care issue or patient concern issue is identified, the Director of Quality Assurance/Utilization Review initiates a Patient Satisfaction Survey Follow-Up Action form which describes the event, incident, or concern and specifies recommendations or corrective actions to be taken (including by whom and by when). This form is returned by an identified person with specific responses and follow-up actions done. Follow-up is monitored and trends identified.

Source: Courtesy of the Visiting Nurse Association of Cleveland, Cleveland, OH.

Exhibit 8-F-3 Patient Survey

Dear Patient:

Have we met your needs?

The staff at the Visiting Nurse Association is dedicated to giving you the best possible care. To do that, we would like your input. Please take a few moments to read this survey. Let us know what you think we are doing well and how we can improve our services. Your responses will be kept strictly confidential, so please feel free to respond frankly.

When completed, seal this self-mailer and drop it in a mail box. Thank you for helping us to serve you better.

Please read each statement carefully and indicate whether you agree or disagree with each statement by checking one box after each statement.

ABOUT YOUR REFERRAL TO HOME CARE

	Strongly Agree	Agree	Do Not Agree	Strongly Disagree
1. I was aware of being referred for home care services.	( )	( )	( )	( )
2. I received my first home care visit soon after referral for service.	( )	( )	( )	( )
3. I understood agency charges and insurance reimbursement.	( )	( )	( )	( )
4. I understood my rights and responsibilities for receiving home care.	( )	( )	( )	( )

Comments: _____

ABOUT YOUR HOME CARE SERVICES

5. I received home care services from the following staff: (Check all that apply.)
( ) Skilled Nursing   ( ) Home Health Aide   ( ) Physical Therapist   ( ) Speech Therapist
( ) Occupational Therapist   ( ) Social Worker   ( ) Nutritionist   ( ) Enterostomal Therapist
( ) Pediatric Nurse   ( ) IV Nurse   ( ) Other; List and Describe: _____

	Strongly Agree	Agree	Do Not Agree	Strongly Disagree
6. The home care staff identified themselves to me by name and title.	( )	( )	( )	( )
7. The home care staff seemed warm, sympathetic and caring.	( )	( )	( )	( )
8. My family and/or I helped plan my home care services.	( )	( )	( )	( )
9. I was satisfied with explanations and instructions about my care.	( )	( )	( )	( )

Comments: _____

continues

Exhibit 8-F-3 continued

	Strongly Agree	Agree	Do Not Agree	Strongly Disagree

ABOUT YOUR DISCHARGE FROM HOME CARE

10. I received help to plan for my needs when services ended. ( ) ( ) ( ) ( )

11. When discharged from home care, I was informed of who to contact regarding health care questions. ( ) ( ) ( ) ( )

Comments: _____

SOME GENERAL QUESTIONS ABOUT HOME CARE

12. In general, how satisfied were you with the care you received from us?
( ) Very satisfied ( ) Satisfied ( ) Dissatisfied ( ) Very Dissatisfied

13. If a family member or friend needed home health services, would you recommend us or another agency?
( ) Recommend the VNA ( ) Recommend another agency   Which one? _____

14. What pleased you most about our home care services? _____

15. In your opinion, what could we do to improve our home care services? _____

Additional comments: _____

Thank you for helping us.

Today's date: _____

Age: _____

( ) Male ( ) Female

Patient's Name: _____

Street Address: _____

City/Zip: _____

Telephone: _____   Dates of service: (from) _____ (to) _____

Name of person completing survey: _____   Relationship to patient: _____

Centre (please check one): ( ) Ohio City ( ) Heights ( ) Lake County

Source: Courtesy of The Visiting Nurse Association of Cleveland, Cleveland, OH.

Exhibit 8-F-4 Patient/Client Satisfaction Survey Report, 2nd Quarter 1989 (For presentation at PAC Meeting on 7/20/89)

	Strongly Agree	Agree	Do Not Agree	Strongly Disagree
1. I was aware of being referred for home care services.				
Skilled Care (n = 113)	69	39	4	1
Special Care (n = 14)	7	7	0	0
All For You				
2. I received my first home care visit soon after referral for service.				
Skilled Care (n = 111)	68	42	1	0
Special Care (n = 14)	8	6	0	0
All For You				
3. I understood agency charges and insurance reimbursement.				
Skilled Care (n = 105)	46	45	8	6
Special Care (n = 13)	4	7	1	1
All For You				
4. I understood my rights and responsibilities.				
Skilled Care (n = 104)	52	45	5	2
Special Care (n = 12)	3	7	1	1
All For You				

5. I received care from: (Skilled Care)

Skilled Nursing	76		
Pediatric Nurse	4		
Nutritionist	2		
HHA	37	PT	30	MSS	13
IV	8	OT	11	Other	0
ET	2	ST	2		

I received care from: (Special Care)

Skilled Nursing	10		
Pediatric Nurse	0		
Nutritionist	2		
Pastoral Care	0		
HHA	8	PT	3	MSS	6
IV	2	OT	2	VOL	2
ET	1	ST	1	Other	0

I received care from: (All For You)

continues

Exhibit 8-F-4 continued

	Strongly Agree	Agree	Do Not Agree	Strongly Disagree
6. The home care staff identified themselves to me by name and title.				
Skilled Care (n = 116)	81	34	1	0
Special Care (n = 13)	9	2	2	0
All For You				
7. The home care staff seemed warm, sympathetic, and caring.				
Skilled Care (n = 114)	85	29	0	0
Special Care (n = 13)	9	4	0	0
All For You				
8. My family and/or I helped plan my home care services.				
Skilled Care (n = 92)	53	32	5	2
Special Care (n = 8)	6	2	0	0
All For You				
9. I was satisfied with explanations and instructions about my care.				
Skilled Care (n = 101)	71	30	0	0
Special Care (n = 10)	7	3	0	0
All For You				
10. I received help to plan for my needs when services ended.				
Skilled Care (n = 70)	42	27	1	0
Special Care (n = 5)	2	2	1	0
All For You				
11. When discharged from home care, I was informed of who to contact regarding health care questions.				
Skilled Care (n = 61)	37	23	1	0
Special Care (n = 5)	2	2	1	0
All For You				

12. In general, how satisfied were you with the care you received from us?

	Very Satisfied	Satisfied	Dissatisfied	Very Dissatisfied
Skilled Care (n=116)	98	18	0	0
Special Care (n=14)	10	3	0	1
All For You				

13. If a family member or friend needed home health services, would you recommend us or another agency?

	Recommend VNA	Recommend Another Agency
Skilled Care (n=112)	110	2
Special Care (n=12)	11	1
All For You		

Centre

Ohio City	41
Heights	81
Lake County	1
Special Care	14
All For You	0

Sex

F	61
M	45

Age

<1 yr.	3
1–9	3
10–19	1
20–29	1
30–39	2
40–49	10
50–59	5
60–69	28
70–79	40
80–89	18
>90	10
Unk.	16

continues

Exhibit 8-F-4 continued

FINDINGS

There were approximately 1387 VNA discharges during the last three months and 137 completed patient satisfaction surveys returned. This approximate 10% return rate is an increase of 3% over last quarter's return rate. 81 of the respondents received care from the Heights Centre staff and 55 received care from the Ohio City Centre staff which includes the Special Care Program. 14 of the respondents were Special Care patients and 123 of the respondents received Skilled Care services. 61 of the respondents were female and 25 were under 60 years of age. 68 of the respondents were between the ages of 60 and 79 years of age and 28 were more than 80 years of age. The median age range was from 70 to 79 years of age and 16 of the respondents did not indicate their age.

110 of 112 skilled care respondents and 11 of 12 special care respondents who answered question #13 indicated that if a family member or a friend needed home health services, they would recommend the VNA over another agency. The one special care patient whose family was dissatisfied with service involved a scheduling error and supervisory follow-up was done.

108 of 113 skilled care patients and 14 of 14 special care patients indicated they were aware of being referred to the VNA for home care services. 110 of 111 skilled care patients and all 14 of the special care patients agreed that the initial visit was timely after they were referred for service. 91 of 105 skilled care patients and 11 of 13 special care patients agreed that they understood agency charges and insurance reimbursement. 97 of 104 skilled care and 10 of 12 special care patients responded that they understood their rights and responsibilities. 115 of 116 skilled care and 11 of 13 special care patients felt the home care staff properly identified themselves and 127 of 127 agreed that the staff seemed warm, sympathetic and caring. 85 of the 92 skilled care and all of the special care patients and/or family members agreed that they participated in the planning of their home care services. All 101 of the skilled care and all 10 of the special care respondents indicated they were satisfied with the explanations and instructions given about their care. 69 of 70 skilled care and 4 of 5 special care patients and/or family members considered themselves helped to plan for needs when services were no longer needed. 60 of 61 skilled care and 4 of 5 special care patients agreed that they were informed of who to contact regarding health care questions after discharged from home care services.

There were 24 skilled care and 6 special care supervisory follow-ups for any indication of dissatisfaction.

Source: Courtesy of the Visiting Nurse Association of Cleveland, Cleveland, OH.

9

Monitoring the Nursing Process

Michael R. Bleich, MPH, RN, CNAA, Vice President for Nursing, Bryan Memorial Hospital, Lincoln, Nebraska, and Healthcare Consultant, Quality Healthcare Resources, Inc., Chicago, Illinois

The nursing process has become the professional, legal, and regulatory framework for judging the efficacy of nursing practice. Monitoring of the nursing process—whether done by nursing peers, regulatory surveyors, or third-party payers—provides insight into the comprehensiveness and impact of nursing care on the patient.

Because of its nature as a problem-solving mechanism, nurses use the nursing process as a guide for clinical problem identification, treatment, and evaluation. This requires the collection and transformation of patient data into clinical judgments. These judgments then stimulate nursing action aimed at meeting the identified physical and emotional needs of patients. Through this dynamic, often spontaneous, and constant interplay among data collection, problem identification, and nursing actions, the nurse is professionally attentive to the nursing process stages of assessment, diagnosis, planning, intervention, and evaluation. The nurse's skill and ability in the use of the nursing process produce problem-focused, goal-driven, and outcome-oriented care.

Monitoring the nursing process takes on professional significance for many reasons. The adequacy of assessments, timeliness of interventions, and successful attainment of desired patient outcomes are but several examples of information that can be gained through a review of the nursing process. This chapter explores these and other facets of the nursing process for clinical review so that insight and direction in improving the quality and appropriateness of patient care may be achieved.

NURSING PROCESS: DEFINITIONS AND FUNCTIONS

The use of the nursing process has continued to vitalize the growth of professional nursing. Recent efforts toward a universal definition of nursing—found in the American Nurses' Association's *Nursing: A Social Policy Statement* (1980), the growing acceptance of nursing diagnoses and the North American Nursing Diagnosis Association's *Diagnostic Taxonomy I* (Lang & Gebbie, 1989), the exploration and clarification of nursing interventions (Bulechek & McCloskey, 1989), and the focus on diagnostic reasoning and clinical judgments (Benner, 1984; Carnevali, 1984)—account for continued depth in understanding the application and use of the nursing process. In order to monitor the nursing process, the current definitions and functions of each process step must be understood.

Assessment

Assessment is the collection of data about the patient obtained during the history/interview, physical examination, and/or laboratory or other diagnostic tests. Assessment data are those aimed at identifying the patient's problems or needs. The assessment is strengthened when a nurse approaches the patient using an organized framework to help assure a holistic view of the patient, or when specialized assessment tools are applied to specific patient situations, such as when initial evidence suggests the presence of clinical problems.

The functions of assessment are to

• generate an organized data base that permits the identification of patient problems or needs

• provide enough knowledge and insight into the patient that individualized planning and interventions are possible

• formulate a base line of clinical information so that a comparison can be made if new problems develop or changes occur in the patient's clinical condition as a result of medical or nursing interventions (Bleich, 1991)

Diagnosis

A nursing diagnosis is a statement that reflects the nurse's clinical judgment and description of a patient's problems or needs in terms where universal meaning results to direct the focus of nursing care. Nursing diagnoses reflect the logical reasoning skills of the nurse.

Nursing diagnoses may be formed using deductive or inductive reasoning skills. Deductive reasoning is used when the nurse knows and recognizes all of the defining characteristics associated with a nursing diagnoses in a presenting clinical situation. If the patient is flushed, is warm to touch, has increased respiratory and heart rates, and has an oral temperature of 101 degrees Fahrenheit, then deductively the nurse concludes that the patient meets the criteria for a nursing diagnosis of hyperthermia.

Inductive reasoning is used when not all of the data have revealed themselves, but when the evidence seems likely enough, based on the past experience of the nurse, that an initial diagnosis and an intervention are warranted. For example, a nurse caring for a postoperative patient may determine from shifts in the patient's blood and central venous pressures, the presence of rales, and restlessness that a fluid volume excess may be developing and thereby take necessary action, even though the same presenting clinical data may also support other patient conditions.

Both deductive and inductive reasoning skills are enhanced through the education and experience of the nurse (Bishop, 1989).

Planning

Once thought of only in terms of a formal document entitled the Nursing Care Plan, planning now includes any documentation that signifies the patient's problem(s), with corresponding expected outcomes and interventions. Planning activities today include documented critical pathways used in case management, predetermined standards of care, computerized care plans, and charting systems that incorporate planning as a part of the documentation routine.

Whatever the mechanism used, the care plan must function to

* consolidate and organize significant patient information (prioritized problems, interventions, and outcomes) into a single resource document or into a consistent retrievable location in the nurses' notes in the medical record
* serve as a communication device between the nurse and the patient
* serve as a communication device between the nurse and the other members of the health care team
* link the nursing process steps of assessment and diagnosis with implementation and evaluation (Bleich, 1991)

Intervention

Interventions are those activities performed by the nurse that provide essential clinical data, or that resolve or alleviate patient problems or needs. Interventions performed by nurses may be either physician- or nurse-initiated (Bulechek & McCloskey, 1989). Physician-initiated interventions are those that assist in the treatment of pathology or medical complications, or that are an iatrogenic residual from medical treatment. Nurse-initiated interventions are those that are designed to treat the patient's human response state, the nature of which is expressed through the nursing diagnosis.

Two common functions are served through the performance of nursing interventions. *Supportive interventions* support the function of providing clinical data needed for ongoing clinical judgments. An example of a supportive intervention is the collection of intake and output, the result of which is clinical data useful for judging the patient's status. *Therapeutic interventions* function to change the patient's human response state, either by altering the condition(s) causing the patient's problem or by enhancing his/her functioning and, therefore, minimizing or diminishing the problem (Griffith-Kenney & Christensen, 1986). Guided imagery is a therapeutic approach to pain management because it diminishes the patient's awareness of the pain. Fluid and bulk intake and increased mobility therapeutically help assure treatment for constipation. Interventions planned for patients should fulfill both supportive and therapeutic functions.

Evaluation

Evaluation calls for another type of clinical judgment. This judgment is used to determine if the patient's problem or need remains status quo, or if it has diminished or increased. Two types of evaluation efforts are required. The first can be called *formative evaluation* because the judgment can be "formed" relatively quickly; formative judgments are associated with observations of the patient's response to interventions. *Summarative evaluations* are derived after observing the patient's condition over a period of time; these judgments relate to the progress shown toward the desired or expected outcome.

Evaluation functions to determine the patient's status as a result of nursing interventions. Interventions that cause the patient additional discomfort or unexpected side effects must be stopped or diminished. Lack of progress toward desired outcomes may require new or increased intervention, assuring the appropriate and effective use of human and material resources.

Evaluation invokes many questions, the answers to which are used to redirect clinical care:

- Is the data base incomplete or inaccurate?
- Is the nursing diagnosis incorrect?
- Is the nursing diagnosis correct, but the outcome unreasonable?
- Is the nursing diagnosis correct, but the intervention wrong, not patient-specific, or in need of increased duration or intensity?

There is no formal language or taxonomy that provides a universal means for describing evaluation judgments. Like assessment judgments, clinical data must support these conclusions.

MONITORING APPROACHES

Monitoring the nursing process effectively depends in large part on knowing what you want to achieve through the review. For example, if the review is to determine whether nurses have adequately assessed and diagnosed patient problems or needs, then monitoring will be limited to a review of assessment data and the resulting nursing diagnoses. If the focus is to determine whether holistic nursing care is being delivered, then nursing diagnoses can be used as indicators to show whether a blend of biophysical, psychological, sociological, and spiritual concerns are being addressed through nursing care. Still another concern may be centered around the timeliness of nursing care from assessment to intervention, information that may signify the priority-setting skills of nurses. These and other approaches to monitoring the nursing process elements are found in Table 9-1.

Two frequent problems are encountered when reviewing the nursing process in patient care records. Often the clinical data are repetitive and dissociated with the diagnosis, intervention, or evaluation to which it is related. Because of this, the data must be considered undifferentiated—that is, they cannot be properly classified into the nursing process framework. This problem occurs when charting systems and agency documentation policies call for information to be segregated onto various chart forms throughout the medical record and again when nurses fail to consciously use the nursing process as a framework for documentation. The second problem is that nurses have only recently been socialized to offer clinical judgments. The growth and acceptance of nursing diagnoses provide nurses with a language to document their assessment judgments. Evaluation judgments remain within the language choice of each nurse; there is no universal language that concisely captures the postintervention status of the patient.

These problems make a review of the nursing process somewhat difficult for evaluators. Evaluators must be skilled in content analysis of patient care records. This means that they must have an excellent grasp of the objectives of the review, the definitions and functions of each nursing process step, the documentation system strengths and weaknesses, and the agency documentation policies and procedures.

Even with this knowledge, the evaluator must recognize that a documentation review does not necessarily mean that the nursing process was not employed in the delivery of patient care. A limitation of documentation review/content analysis is that it demonstrates only whether or not the nursing process was documented; observed clinical practice and dialogue with nurses may be needed to fully judge the extent to which nursing process guides clinical practice.Regardless, documentation of the nursing process is becoming an industry standard for determining whether reimbursement should be paid, whether care was delivered in a legally acceptable manner, and so on.

Table 9-1 Approaches to Monitoring the Nursing Process Elements

Aspect of Care	Focus of the Monitor	Sample Criteria
1. Adequacy of initial assessment	To review whether initial assessments are completed in a timely manner and contain information sufficient to identify patient problems/needs, establish expected outcomes and interventions that are patient-specific, and establish a base line for future assessments	1. The assessment is completed within the defined unit time frame. 2. The assessment is completed by qualified personnel. 3. The assessment includes information related to the patient's • current medical history • past medical history • biophysical dimension (vital signs, physical examination results) • psychological dimension • sociological dimension • spiritual dimension
2. Adequacy of specialized assessments	To review whether specialized assessments are conducted when specific patient problems are evident and to examine the accuracy and thoroughness of these assessments	1. A specialized assessment is completed and documented when a deviation (e.g., cardiovascular abnormality) is noted. 2. Specialized assessments are recorded according to the specialty unit protocol. 3. Cardiovascular assessment, when indicated, contains the following elements: • apical rate and rhythm • heart sounds/murmurs • peripheral pulses • pain • activity, etc.
3. Adequacy of nursing diagnosis	To review whether nursing diagnoses are derived from the assessment data and whether clinical priorities are reflected.	1. Health pattern deviations result in a stated nursing diagnosis. 2. Nursing diagnoses are stated in a problem and etiology format. 3. Nursing diagnoses reflect clinical priorities (i.e., life-threatening physiological deviations over other conditions/human response states).

continues

Table 9-1 continued

Aspect of Care	Focus of the Monitor	Sample Criteria
Adequacy of nursing diagnosis (cont.)		4. Clinical problems are clearly stated when nursing diagnoses are not used or do not reflect the patient's needs.
4. Provision of holistic care	To assure that nursing assessment, diagnoses, planning, interventions, and evaluation reflect concern for the total person.	1. Assessment reflects data from each human dimension: • biophysical • psychological • sociological • spiritual 2. Nursing diagnoses are varied to reflect holistic needs. 3. Specific interventions are designed and implemented to treat the whole person. 4. Evaluation shows attention to each stated problem/expected outcome/intervention.
5. Prioritized planning	To review the adequacy of care planning and the clinical priorities of the nurse.	1. Life-threatening physiological problems are listed before other problems. 2. In the absence of life-threatening problems, the reason for seeking health care is addressed. 3. Patient/family priorities are considered as input in developing the plan of care.
6. Adequacy of interventions	To review whether both supportive and therapeutic interventions are carried out, considering the patient's sociocultural history.	1. Supportive interventions are documented. 2. Therapeutic interventions are documented and include • who performed the intervention • what was done • how long it was performed • whether it is patient-specific
7. Adequacy of evaluation	To review whether formative and summarizing evaluations are carried out.	1. Patient response to the intervention is noted. 2. Patient progress toward expected outcomes is noted: • response shows progress, retrogression, or status quo • assessment, plans, and interventions are expanded or adjusted, as appropriate • discharge planning reflects current patient status

Joint Commission and Professional Nurse Chart Review

Throughout the 1980s, the Joint Commission on Accreditation of Healthcare Organizations, through its nursing service standards, has emphasized the use of the nursing process. As of January 1991, a chapter that addresses the delivery of nursing care throughout the organization was put into effect (Joint Commission, 1990). As in the past, an emphasis on the use of the nursing process to deliver nursing care remains.

The revised Joint Commission nursing care standards make two primary changes regarding the use of the nursing process (Joint Commission, 1990). The first change recognizes that a number of qualified health care providers may contribute to the initial history/data base, whereas, in the past, this function remained within the exclusive domain of the registered nurse. Through defined standards of practice, each organization can now determine if other roles, such as licensed practical nurses or mental health technicians, should contribute to the initial data base. Still, the registered nurse must determine if the data base is complete and draw the nursing diagnoses or patient problems from the information (Accreditation Clinic, 1990). A checklist of elements to review for evidence of the nursing process is found in Exhibit 9-1.

The second change relates to how the nursing plan of care is documented. In the past, the Joint Commission required the presence of a single document entitled the nursing care plan. Now this plan can be included in a variety of schemata as long as it is retrievable and evidenced within the medical record. As mentioned earlier, this gives organizations the flexibility to document the nursing care plan through critical pathways, through standards of patient care and practice, within documentation systems, and so on.

Remaining unchanged in the new nursing care standards are the scope of the initial assessment, the presence of a retrievable plan of care, the documentation of nursing interventions, and a review of the patient's response to these interventions. A review of closed medical records will continue to be one way that surveyors review the nursing process. Other mechanisms may evolve that include a review of the nursing care being delivered to hospitalized patients through staff and patient interviews (Patterson, 1990).

DOCUMENTATION SYSTEMS: RETRIEVING NURSING PROCESS DATA

Retrieval of nursing process information from the medical record requires some knowledge about the various types of medical record systems that are in common use. Once narrative charting was the standard fare for recording nursing observa-

Exhibit 9-1 Documentation Checklist of Elements To Review for Evidence of the Nursing Process

	Yes	No

1. Assessment includes:
  –biophysical factors
  –psychosocial factors
  –environmental factors
  –self-care factors
  –educational factors
  –discharge planning factors		

2. Initial and ongoing assessments are recorded.		
3. Nursing diagnoses/patient care needs are evident.		
4. Interventions are identified and carried out to meet patient care needs.		
5. The patient's response to interventions are noted.		
6. The outcomes of care are recorded.		
7. The degree to which patients can manage self care is recorded.		
8. Collaboration with other health care disciplines is evident, as indicated.		
9. Patient education is provided throughout the hospital stay, as indicated.		
10. The patient and family is included in clinical decisions regarding care.		

Source: Data from *Accreditation Manual for Hospitals*, vol. 1 (pp. 131–132) by Joint Commission on Accreditation of Healthcare Organizations, 1991.

tions and interventions, but with the growing use of the nursing process as a method for practicing nursing, other systems have developed. Computerized documentation systems, problem-oriented systems, Focus charting, and PIE charting are examples of new process-oriented documentation systems. Each system attempts to organize the increasingly large amounts of clinical data that nurses are responsible for recording.

The fact that each of these new systems reflects the nursing process is an aid to understanding their similarities and differences.

- Each charting system includes opportunities for recording nursing assessments. Usually these opportunities include a comprehensive initial data base, followed by ongoing assessments completed and recorded based on the type of health care agency, clinical unit, and/or patient condition. The ongoing assessment is documented within the context of the clinical notes or may be on special flow records that allow the nurse to compare patient data.

- Care planning is recorded on a separate form that serves as the basis for charting, or it may be included as a part of the construct within a charting system.

- Interventions of a routine nature are often recorded on flow sheets or graphic records. Interventions directly related to the patient's plan of care most often are recorded in the clinical notes. Special nursing interventions, such as patient teaching, may appear on forms specially designed to show the depth and breadth of instruction and usually allow space for documenting the patient's response to the intervention.

- The evaluation of the patient's response to interventions generally appears as a narrative entry following the recorded intervention. Sometimes flow charts will contain space for recording the patient's response to interventions; for example, a pain management flow record might display the intervention and patient's response to the intervention in such a manner that evaluation judgments of patient progress are possible. Finally, the patient's progress toward meeting the expected outcomes are recorded either as free text or on special forms, such as transfer or discharge summaries.

Following are summaries of documentation systems that incorporate the use of the nursing process. The comments serve to guide a reviewer to evidence of the nursing process.

PIE System

PIE is an acronym that refers to documenting the patient's Problems, Interventions, and Evaluations. The system is based on initial and ongoing assessments of each patient (each shift), the formulation of a problem list (preferably stated as nursing diagnoses), and the recording of clinical notes on each relevant problem. Each problem is given a number, which is entered in the notes. The interventions are recorded next to the problem, followed by an evaluation comment noting the patient's response/progress each shift, and are summarized at transfer or discharge (Siegrest, Dettor, & Stocks, 1985).

Focus System

Focus charting allows the nurse to document, in a Focus column, the focus of his or her nursing care—stated as a symptom, a significant hospital event, or a nursing diagnosis. In an adjacent column, the nurse then records the associated *data* (either assessment or evaluative), *action* (the nursing interventions), and *response* (the patient response or progress) (Lampe, 1985).

Problem-Oriented Systems

The problem-oriented system uses a construct known as SOAP or, in its extended format, SOAPIER. This acronym stands for Subjective and Objective data, Assessment, Plan, Intervention, Evaluation, and Revision. In the extended form, the S and O combine to provide the clinical data needed for the assessment (nursing diagnosis). Interventions and evaluation follow, including any revisions that may be required to advance the patient's care (Lindberg, Hunter, & Kruszewski, 1983). In its abbreviated form, there is a tendency to document the evaluation of the patient's response to an intervention under the assessment, thereby confusing the nursing process functions of assessment and evaluation.

Computerized Systems

Many computerized systems are now available to assist nurses with charting, including some at the bedside (Albarado, McCall & Thrane, 1990; Herring & Rochman, 1990; Romano, McCormick, & McNeely, 1982). Typically, these computerized systems are ideal for documenting the patient's assessment data and for generating a plan of care. Many systems are designed to document interventions driven by the care plan. Unless the nurse enters free text, many computer systems are unable to reflect the evaluation phase of the nursing process, even though computers have the capability of tracking and trending data that can be used as an adjunct to deriving a nursing judgment of the patient's status over a period of time.

Narrative Systems

Although not a process-cuing system, narrative charting does not prohibit the nurse from recording the nursing process, although the steps of the process may not be as evident. Narrative systems begin with a patient assessment and are dependent on the use of a care plan. The notes encountered in narrative charting tend to be a mix of nursing observations (assessment or evaluation) and interventions. The patient's response to interventions may be recorded, but the nurse is not cued to enter evaluation responses. Because there is no formal place to document the nursing diagnosis/patient problem, this information is the most likely to be absent from the record (Fischbach & Bleich, 1991).

A. The chain is complete when all nursing process elements can be identified and linked together.

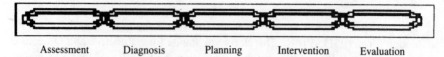

Assessment   Diagnosis   Planning   Intervention   Evaluation

1. A chain is initiated each time a clinical problem is evident and all of the data elements that precede and proceed are evident.
2. Track each chain throughout the patient care record.

B. The chain is interrupted when only the patient problem or another singular element of the nursing process is present *or* when the nursing process elements are fragmented and cannot be connected.

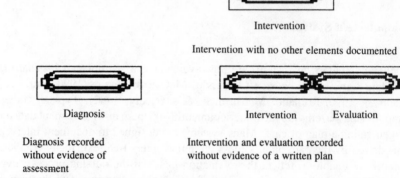

Intervention

Intervention with no other elements documented

Diagnosis   Intervention   Evaluation

Diagnosis recorded   Intervention and evaluation recorded
without evidence of   without evidence of a written plan
assessment

1. Content must be reviewed and related to other data.
2. The types of data missing are totaled to determine the frequency of missing links.

C. The chain is incomplete when the process has not been carried out to its fullest extent.

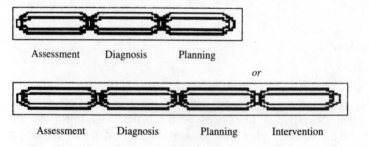

Assessment   Diagnosis   Planning

or

Assessment   Diagnosis   Planning   Intervention

1. Determine the number of incomplete chains.
2. Determine the adequacy at discharge planning and/or at follow-up to achieve completion of the process.

Figure 9-1 Examining Chains of the Nursing Process. *Source:* Adapted from J. Baumgart (1978). *Developing an instrument for measuring the nursing process.* Unpublished master's thesis, University of Illinois.

IMPLICATIONS FOR PRACTICE

To document the nursing process, one must first recognize that the nursing process is linear; that is, each step is an outgrowth of the other steps. Documentation must show the relationship of assessment to diagnosis, diagnosis to intervention, and intervention to evaluation (see Figure 9-1). Charting systems based on the nursing process make these relationships possible.

Contrary to popular belief, everything that the nurse observes, processes, and acts on cannot always be fully understood or comprehended within a tour of duty. To aid in the documentation of the nursing process, the nurse focuses on the patient's reason for seeking care, the nature of the agency and/or unit where care is delivered, and the standards for observations and documentation within the organization.

The novice nurse may lack experience in drawing deductive or inductive conclusions about the patient's needs and, therefore, have problems in recording the nursing process. The expert nurse may act out of such a strong sense of intuition that converting intuition back into process may create an equal documentation challenge (Benner, 1984; Miller, 1989).

While these challenges will always exist, the fact remains that nursing is a client-centered profession. As such, nurses are expected to use their knowledge and skills, coupled with their knowledge of socially ascribed nursing roles, to ascertain a patient's needs and to provide services based on these needs. Monitoring the nursing process helps generate and expand nursing knowledge and subsequently improve practice.

Monitoring the nursing process makes it possible for individual nurses to gain insight into their practice and can serve as a type of peer review. Agencies that review the nursing process can make inferences about the quality of nursing care, nursing role activities, patient care delivery systems, and continuity of care.

CONCLUSION

Nursing is growing as an art and a science. The nursing process provides a structure for examining the scientific, problem-driven, and goal-driven focuses of nursing in meeting the needs of patients. Furthermore, this process is beneficial for expanding nursing knowledge and for achieving social accountability. Monitoring the nursing process gives individual nurses and agencies critical information about the nature and quality of care being delivered.

REFERENCES

Accreditation Clinic. (1990). *Joint Commission Perspectives, 10*(4), 8–9.

Albarado, R.S., McCall, V., & Thrane, J.M. (1990). Computerized nursing documentation. *Nursing Management, 21*(7), 64–65.

American Nurses' Association. (1980). *Nursing: A social policy statement.* Kansas City, MO: Author.

Baumgart, J. (1978). *Developing an instrument for measuring the nursing process.* Unpublished master's thesis, University of Illinois.

Benner, P. (1984). *From novice to expert: Excellence and power in clinical nursing practice.* Menlo Park, CA: Addison-Wesley.

Bishop, S.M. (1989). Logical reasoning. In A. Marriner-Tomey (Ed.), *Nursing theorists and their work* (2nd ed.). St. Louis: C.V. Mosby.

Bleich, M.R. (1991). Documenting the nursing process. In F. Fischbach (Ed.), *Documenting care: Communications, nursing process, and documentation standards.* Philadelphia: F.A. Davis.

Bulechek, G.M., & McCloskey, J.C. (1989). Nursing interventions: Treatments for potential nursing diagnoses. In R.M. Carroll-Johnson (Ed.), *Classification of nursing diagnoses.* Philadelphia: J.B. Lippincott.

Carnevali, D.L., Mitchell, P.H., Woods, N.F., & Tanner, C.A. (1984). *Diagnostic reasoning in nursing.* Philadelphia: J.B. Lippincott.

Fischbach, F., & Bleich, M. (1991). Documentation systems and the nursing process. In F. Fischbach (Ed.), *Documenting care: Communications, nursing process, and documentation standards.* Philadelphia: F.A. Davis.

Griffith-Kenney, J.W., & Christensen, P.J. (1986). *Nursing process: Applications to theories, frameworks, and models.* St. Louis: C.V. Mosby.

Herring, D., & Rochman, R. (1990). A closer look at bedside terminals. *Nursing Management, 21*(7), 54–61.

Joint Commission on Accreditation of Healthcare Organizations. (1990). *The new standards for nursing care* (2nd ed.). Oakbrook Terrace, IL: Author.

Lampe, S. (1985). Focus charting: Streamlining documentation. *Nursing Management, 16*(7), 43–46.

Lang, N.M., & Gebbie, K. (1989). Nursing taxonomy: NANDA and ANA joint venture toward ICD–10CM. In R.M. Carroll-Johnson (Ed.), *Classification of nursing diagnoses.* Philadelphia: J.B. Lippincott.

Lindberg, J., Hunter, M., & Kruszewski, A. (1983). *Introduction to person-centered nursing.* Philadelphia: J.B. Lippincott.

Miller, V.G. (1989). Analysis and intuition: The need for both in nursing education. *Journal of Nursing Education, 28*(2), 84–86.

Patterson, C. (1990, July). *Preparing for compliance: The new Joint Commission nursing care standards.* Satellite teleconference. American Hospital Association.

Romano, C., McCormick, K.A., & McNeely, L.D. (1982). Nursing documentation: A model for a computerized data base. *Advances in Nursing Science,* 43–56.

Siegrest, L.M., Dettor, R.E., & Stocks, B. (1985). The PIE system: Complete planning and documentation of nursing care. *Quality Review Bulletin,* 186–189.

10

Using Statistics in Quality Assurance

Paul A. Reichelt, PhD, Associate Professor, Department of Administrative Studies in Nursing, College of Nursing, University of Illinois at Chicago, Chicago, Illinois

> Statistical thinking will one day be as necessary for efficient citizenship as the ability to read and write.
>
> —H.G. Wells

Like many of H.G. Wells' predictions about the intriguing future he foresaw in his science fiction writings, his comment about statistics is true today in general and in particular when working in quality assurance (QA). Fortunately for nursing, the correct use of statistics has been an important aspect of clinical practice since Florence Nightingale's seminal work during the Crimean War. In fact, a recent book (Jaffe & Spirer, 1987) containing a large assortment of examples of misuses of statistics cites Nightingale's work as an excellent example of the *proper* use of statistics.

Statistics is an important QA tool because it encompasses a large variety of methods for presenting, summarizing, and analyzing data. Because all nurses require feedback about the quality of patient care being delivered, it follows that all nurses will have continuing contact with statistical procedures either as creators or as users of QA data or, most probably, as both. This chapter will not attempt to condense a standard statistics book into a few pages of text likely to trigger an attack of statistics anxiety. Rather, the approach taken here is to present statistics as a very powerful communication technique that can be used by anyone to improve the quality of decision making. The emphasis is on the logic behind the most commonly used types of statistics as a way to guide the reader to the formulas contained in such statistics texts as Hays (1988), Knapp (1985), and Volicer (1984). Given that most data are currently analyzed using software run on computers ranging from laptops to mainframes, one may never even directly refer to the formulas. Regardless of how the calculations are performed, the most important concepts to be aware of are those that allow one to understand how statistics can serve as an aid to the interpretation of nursing QA data.

MEASUREMENT AND STATISTICAL PROCEDURES

Before any statistical procedures can be selected, the data must be collected. Deciding what QA data to collect is, of course, a nursing decision, rather than a statistical decision. Only at the point of deciding how to collect the data do nursing and statistics interface. The first issue is how to ensure that accurate data are collected. This refers to the reliability and validity of the data. If inaccurate data are collected, either because the data collector has not been properly trained to use the measurement instrument or because the instrument itself (whether the latest piece of high technology or the very common paper-and-pencil tool) is poorly constructed or calibrated, usually little can be done statistically to fully overcome the measurement shortcomings. The interested reader will find thoughtful discussions of approaches for ensuring the reliability and validity of nursing data contained in most nursing research textbooks and in volumes specifically concerned with measurement issues (e.g., Waltz, Strickland, & Lenz, 1984).

Another measurement issue to keep in mind when calculating or interpreting statistics concerns the level of measurement inherent in the data collection procedures used to measure the patient characteristics or other variables under study. Four levels of measurement are generally described in the literature: nominal, ordinal, interval, and ratio.

The nominal scale of measurement is simply the classification of patients into specified categories or values of the variable when there is no necessary relationship among the values. A common clinical example is the variable blood type. Type A blood is simply different than type B blood; it is not better or worse, more or less, etc. If numerals are assigned to the different categories of a nominal scale, such as to a list of nursing diagnoses, these numerals are merely symbols that do not have the quantitative meaning usually attributed to such symbols; that is, these numerals are not numbers upon which arithmetic operations can be performed.

An ordinal scale of measurement is the next higher level of measurement in that it provides more information about the variable or characteristic being measured. With an ordinal scale, the different values or categories are ranked in terms of an ordered relationship. If a QA study asked patients whether they were very dissatisfied, dissatisfied, satisfied, or very satisfied with the nursing care they had received, clearly a patient who answered "very satisfied" has greater patient satisfaction than does a patient who answered "satisfied." However, the magnitude of that greater satisfaction is not specified by such an ordinal scale.

Interval and ratio scales represent the addition of further information to the measurement process because the distances between any two values on these scales are of equal size. A patient who weighs 160 pounds is the same amount heavier than a patient who weighs 150 pounds as that second patient is heavier than a third patient who weighs 140 pounds. These values are true numbers. The difference between interval and ratio scales is that a ratio scale has a true zero point, while an interval scale does not. Weight is a ratio scale because its zero point represents the total absence of weight. Patient temperatures measured in degrees Fahrenheit or centigrade are an interval scale, but not a ratio scale, because their zero points are arbitrary and do not represent the total absence of heat.

A helpful measurement strategy is to use data collection instruments that result in the highest level of measurement possible for the variables of interest. Data measured at a higher level of measurement can always be reduced to a lower level, if appropriate, but the reverse is not true. More informative statistical procedures can be performed using exact patient age in years, for example, and the data can subsequently be collapsed into age groups for other presentation purposes. But if the data are collected only in terms of age categories, the application of certain useful statistical procedures is not possible. The importance of the level of measurement distinctions for statistics is that different procedures make different assumptions about the type of information represented by the data being analyzed. This will be discussed as different types of statistics are presented.

TABULAR DATA PRESENTATION

Descriptive statistics are those procedures designed to organize a set of data in a concise manner so that the information can be more readily communicated. This is accomplished through the use of tabular and graphic presentations and through the calculation of summary statistics. Of these methods, tables are probably the most frequently used technique for presenting quality assurance and other nursing data.

The purpose of a table is illustrated by the following example where data on the nominal-level variable of medical diagnosis have been collected for 23 patients receiving venous therapy at home (Barget & Zink, 1989). Presenting this information by listing 23 patient numbers followed by the diagnosis would obviously be cumbersome and would not facilitate the description of the 23 individuals as a group. Organizing the data into a frequency distribution, as shown in Table 10-1, is more concise and allows the reader to quickly determine the existence of commonalities in medical diagnosis among the patients receiving venous therapy. The three columns of this table present the values (categories) of the primary medical diagnosis variable, the absolute frequency or count of how many times each value occurs in this sample, and the relative frequency with which each value occurs, which is a percentage calculated as the absolute frequency divided by the total.

A reader looking at a table can easily see the range of values and the most prevalent values. Tables and the columns within them should be clearly labeled, and the total size of the data set being presented should be indicated.

When a large number of different values exist for the variable being presented, even a table will quickly become rather cumbersome. This problem can be

Table 10-1 Primary Medical Diagnoses of Patients Receiving Venous Therapy at Home

Medical Diagnosis	Frequency	Percent
Infection	7	30.4
Cancer	7	30.4
Osteomyelitis	4	17.4
Cellulitis	2	8.7
Malnutrition	1	4.3
Bowel obstruction	1	4.3
Scleraderma	1	4.3
Total	23	99.8

Note: Percentages do not total 100.0 due to rounding.

Source: Adapted from "Evaluation of Clinical Indicators in IV Home Care" by C.D. Barget and M.R. Zink, 1989, *Journal of Nursing Quality Assurance, 3*(3), p. 68. Copyright 1989 by Aspen Publishers, Inc.

overcome by using a grouped frequency table where the different values are organized into a smaller set of groups of values and the frequency of each grouping or class interval is presented. For example, if the 23 patients from Table 10-1 were each a different number of years old, the 23 different values for the ratio-level variable of age might be organized into five 10-year class intervals:

20–29
30–39
40–49
50–59
60–69

The addition of frequency and percentage columns will readily convert this list of class intervals into an easy-to-read, grouped frequency table. Three guidelines should be kept in mind when constructing class intervals.

1. The intervals should be mutually exclusive so that any given value fits into only one of them. Class intervals for age such as 20–30, 30–40, etc., are incorrect because the intervals overlap, and it is not clear where an age such as 30 should be placed.
2. The set of class intervals should be exhaustive so that there is an appropriate interval to contain every one of the different values.
3. Intervals of equal width make a table easier to read.

Tables can be easily expanded to present more than one set of data. If the 23 patients described in Table 10-1 were from community *A*, and an additional group of 27 patients from community *B* who were receiving venous therapy at home was also of interest, a pair of columns inserted for community *B* patients would quickly result in Table 10-2. To avoid a cluttered look in this expanded table, the frequency column heading has been changed to *n* (commonly used number), and the % sign is used for the relative frequency column.

This expanded table provides a good illustration of the function served by the use of percentages when comparing data from groups of unequal size. Although there are equal numbers of patients with osteomyelitis in both communities, such patients comprise a larger proportion of the community *A* group. The use of relative frequencies allows the direct comparison of different-sized groups by using the same base of 100 percent, whereas a comparison of the absolute frequencies can lead to an erroneous conclusion. When using percentages, it is important to keep in mind the total size of the group under consideration. While 75 percent sounds like a large figure, it is still only three patients if the total group size is four.

GRAPHIC DATA PRESENTATION

In addition to tables, graphic presentations are another excellent device for displaying QA data. Various types of bar charts, such as Figure 10-1, are a frequently encountered type of pictorial display in the nursing literature (Robertson & DeCampli, 1988). Absolute or relative frequencies are usually

---

Table 10-2 Primary Medical Diagnoses of Community *A* and Community *B* Patients Receiving Venous Therapy at Home

Medical Diagnosis	Community A		Community B	
	n	%	*n*	%
Infection	7	30.4	8	29.6
Cancer	7	30.4	9	33.3
Osteomyelitis	4	17.4	4	14.8
Cellulitis	2	8.7	3	11.1
Malnutrition	1	4.3	1	3.7
Bowel obstruction	1	4.3	2	7.4
Scleraderma	1	4.3	0	0.0
Total	23	99.8	27	99.9

Note: Percentages do not total 100.0 due to rounding.

Source: Adapted from "Evaluation of Clinical Indicators in IV Home Care" by C.D. Barget and M.R. Zink, 1989, *Journal of Nursing Quality Assurance, 3*(3), p. 68. Copyright 1989 by Aspen Publishers, Inc.

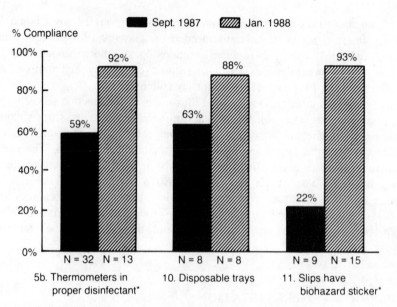

Figure 10-1 Hospital Summary of Randomly Selected Patients Requiring Specific Infection Control Practices—Patient Environment. *Source:* Adapted from ''Infection Control Rounds: A Method for Evaluating Safety'' by M.R. Robertson and P.D. DeCampli, 1988, *Journal of Nursing Quality Assurance, 3*(1), p. 50. Copyright 1988 by Aspen Publishers, Inc.

*Figure categories reflect criteria numbers listed on the Monitoring and Evaluation Tool: Infection Control.

plotted on the vertical axis, and categories are shown along the horizontal axis. When the categories on the horizontal axis are continuous numerical intervals such as patient age, rather than a set of distinct groups such as diagnoses, the graph is called a *histogram*. Graphs are especially useful for displaying such comparisons as changes over time, as shown in Figure 10-1, and differences between groups. Table 10-2 can be readily converted into a graph by plotting percentages on the vertical axis and medical diagnosis categories on the horizontal axis, and by using one bar for community *A* and another for community *B* for each diagnosis. With seven diagnostic categories, a total of 14 bars would be necessary to display the data from Table 10-2. This might look too visually cluttered and is a reminder that tables can often accommodate more data than graphs. However, graphs have greater visual impact and are easier to read at a distance when using posters or projected slides/overheads to present data. As with tables, graphs need to be clearly labeled so that they can be readily comprehended without having to refer to any accompanying text.

The frequency scale often used on the vertical axis of bar charts may be replaced by any other useful scale such as infection rate or number of analgesic doses administered. The bars can be replaced by data points connected by a line to create the often-seen line graph that can easily display multiple data sets, such as one line for females and another for males. A circle representing 100 percent can be sliced into segments denoting proportions of the total to create the familiar pie chart, perhaps showing the percentages of a hospital's clientele funded by different payment sources. The variety of graphs that can be devised is limited only by the imagination and the requirement that they clearly communicate the information contained in the data without distortion or confusing clutter. Distortion can inadvertently occur as a result of such common mistakes as using equal spacing along an axis to represent unequal-sized intervals and comparing costs for different years without adjusting the dollar values for inflation.

MEASURES OF CENTRAL TENDENCY

In addition to tables and graphs, a set of data can be summarized by calculating numerical descriptors. The statistics most commonly used for this purpose are the various measures of central tendency and dispersion. Measures of central tendency are numbers used to describe the center of a distribution of data. The arithmetic mean or average is one such statistic. It is simply the sum of all the scores divided by the number of scores that were summed. It is the center of the data distribution in the sense that the total amount by which some scores in the distribution are greater than the mean is equal to the total amount by which other scores are less than the mean. Caution should be exercised when interpreting a mean based on a distribution that contains one or more extreme values, especially when the total number of scores in the set of data is small. For example, if the ages in years of six patients are 21, 23, 23, 26, 28, and 82, the mean is the sum of 203 divided by 6, which equals 33.8 years. In a situation such as this, the mean is moved toward the extreme score and will not represent the average of the distribution in terms of being a typical score. A mean for a sample of scores is symbolized by M or $\bar{X}$ (pronounced X bar) and may be calculated for interval- and ratio-level data.

Although clear definitions of nominal, ordinal, interval, and ratio scales of measurement were presented earlier in this chapter, the measurement tools often used in nursing and many other disciplines produce data that seem to fall in between the ordinal and interval categories. For example, when patients are presented with a Likert-type scale where they are asked to use a five- or seven-point response scale to indicate the extent of their agreement or disagreement with statements about the nursing care they have received, the resulting data are certainly ordinal, but may not contain exactly equal intervals. A long history of practical applications has demonstrated that such data can generally be treated as if they were interval data when deciding what statistical procedures to use.

A second measure of central tendency is the median (Md or Mdn), which is the middle score of a distribution when the values for all the persons being measured on the variable are arranged in order from low to high. When there is an odd number of measurements, the median is the actual middle score in the ordered set of measurements. When there is an even number of measurements, the median is the mean of the two middle scores (i.e., the median is not one of the actual scores in the distribution). The median is the center of the distribution in the sense that the numbers of scores above and below the median are equal. Unlike the mean, the median is not as affected by extreme values in the distribution, which is why it is frequently used for variables where extreme values, such as patient age and average length of stay for patients in a particular DRG (diagnosis related group), can occur. The median for the six patient ages previously presented is 24.5 years, the average of the two middle scores of 23 and 26. A median may be calculated for ordinal- or higher-level data.

The mode is the last measure of central tendency. It is the value that occurs most frequently in a set of scores, and so is the center of the distribution only in terms of frequency of occurrence. The mode of the six patient ages is 23 years. A distribution can also have no mode (all the scores are different), be bimodal (two scores occur with the same frequency), or be multimodal (three or more modes exist). The mode can be used with any level of measurement, but is typically used as the sole measure of central tendency only for nominal-level data.

MEASURES OF DISPERSION

Once the central tendency of a distribution has been described using one or more of the three statistics just discussed, the distribution should be further summarized by calculating its variability. Measures of dispersion or variability describe the extent of the scattering of scores within the distribution. The simplest measure of dispersion is the range, which is defined as the largest value in the distribution minus the smallest value. Because the range is calculated using only the two scores that form the boundaries of the distribution, the range can be dramatically affected by an extreme score (sometimes called an *outlier*) in the data set. For example, if the length of stay for five patients is 3, 2, 4, 3, and 5 days, the range is 3 days. If a patient is added to the group whose length of stay is 12 days, the range becomes 10 days. A common interpretation error is to look at a range and to assume that scores are distributed throughout the range. As this example illustrates, large parts of the distribution between the high and low scores may be empty. It is also quite possible to have the same range for distributions that are quite dissimilar. For example, length of stay scores of 2, 9, 11, 10, and 12 days also have a range of 10. A range may be calculated for ordinal- or higher-level data.

The variance and standard deviation are two forms of a measure of dispersion that provide greater information about a set of data because unlike the range, which considers only the two endpoints of the distribution, these two statistics are calculated using all the scores and measure the degree to which the scores deviate from the mean of the distribution. Because the mean is the exact center of a distribution, the sum of the deviations of the scores from the mean, and thus the average deviation, is always zero. Therefore, the variance (symbolized for a sample as s^2) is defined as the average of the squared deviations of the scores from the mean. Taking the square root of the variance results in the standard deviation (s) which is easier to use because it is the same unit of measurement as the original data. The variance and standard deviation can be calculated for interval and ratio data, and as was noted previously, such statistics are typically also used for ordinal data that approximate an interval scale.

A distribution of scores resulting from such measurement procedures can be succinctly summarized by reporting the mean and the standard deviation. Referring back to Table 10-2 for an example, the mean number of nursing visits for the 23 patients in community A might be 12.0 with a standard deviation of 1.9 visits, while the statistics for community B patients might be a mean of 13.4 visits with a standard deviation of 4.2. The larger mean for community B reveals that on average those patients had more nursing visits, and the larger standard deviation indicates greater variability in number of visits among those patients than among community A patients. In other words, the nursing visits scores are more closely clustered around the mean in the community A distribution than in the community B distribution. Additional statistics can also be reported, such as the ranges (specifying the endpoints of the distributions) and the modes (indicating the most common numbers of nursing visits).

RELATIVE FREQUENCY

Percentages or relative frequencies have already been discussed in the context of their use in tables and graphs, where it was noted that they allow for direct comparison among groups composed of different numbers of individuals by using a common base of 100 percent. A second type of comparison frequently made using percentages concerns change over time. Figure 10-1 contains examples showing changes in the percentage of compliance from September 1987 to January 1988 for three criteria. Percentage of change is calculated as

$$\frac{\text{Final value} - \text{initial value}}{\text{Initial value}} \times 100$$

This calculates out to a 56 percent increase in percentage of compliance for the criterion of thermometers being properly handled. This is obviously a positive outcome, which is the correct conclusion to draw from the data. If percentages were not used to make this comparison where the number of patients is different for the two time periods, the absolute frequencies could be easily misinterpreted as pointing to a negative outcome; that is, the number of correctly handled thermometers decreased from 19 (59 percent of 32 patients) to 12 (92 percent of 13 patients).

A common type of confusion that arises when discussing changes in percentages can be illustrated by looking at a familiar political example for variety. If a sales tax is increased from 4 percent to 5 percent, politicians will typically talk about the fact that the tax rate has only increased by one percentage point. However, taxpayers counting their change at the store will quickly realize that they are paying 25 percent more sales tax.

Although relative frequencies make it easy to compare groups of different sizes, the base on which percentages are calculated cannot be ignored. Earlier, a caution was voiced about interpreting percentages based on very small groups. Another situation where group size is important occurs when percentages are being averaged. Unless each percentage is based on exactly the same size group, each must be weighted by the total on which it is based. To accomplish this, each of the absolute frequencies is summed, and this sum is divided by the sum of the totals on which the frequencies are based. For the thermometer example above, the average percentage of correctly handled thermometers during the entire time period of the QA study is $(19 + 12) \div (32 + 13) = 69\%$. It is not appropriate to add 59 percent to 92 percent and divide by 2 because the two groups used to calculate those two percentages are of different size and the larger group must be given greater weight when calculating the average. This same consideration applies to means. To average means, each mean must be weighted by the size of the group it represents, except for the special case where all the groups are the same size and, therefore, each mean deserves equal weight in calculating the average mean.

INFERENTIAL STATISTICS

In addition to descriptive statistics that may be used any time data are collected, the realm of statistics includes another major aspect that is often useful for analyzing QA data. This aspect is known as inferential statistics because it is composed of a large number of procedures that allow one to make inferences about a larger population of data based on a smaller sample drawn from that population. This is a very efficient tool for decision making because it permits the formulation of statements about the population of interest with a known degree of accuracy without spending the time and resources necessary to study the entire population. The value of inferential statistics is dramatically illustrated by the pervasive example of national public opinion polls where a sample of only about 2,000 residents is used to gauge the feelings of the entire American population.

In order for inferential statistics to result in accurate inferences about the population of interest, the prime prerequisite is that the data be collected from a representative sample drawn from that population. The best way to assure representativeness is to use random sampling procedures. These procedures are based on probability theory in order to eliminate selection bias during sampling so that a representative sample can be achieved.

For example, a nursing QA study might begin by defining the population of interest as all patients treated in the hospital during the previous 12 months who required intravenous (IV) therapy. This population will be rather large for many hospitals, and considerable time and expense would be incurred collecting data from all these patient records. However, using a table of random numbers or a computer-generated list of random numbers, a simple random sample can be easily selected so that each patient in the population has an equal chance of being included in the sample. Other probability sampling designs might also be used, depending on the focus of the QA study. One possibility is to stratify the population and then select a random sample from each stratum. The population might be divided into those patients who had central IV lines and those patients who had peripheral IV lines so that a sample could be drawn from each of these two subpopulations or strata. Nursing research textbooks contain discussions of various probability and nonprobability sampling methods, and further detail can be found in sampling texts and the sampling sections of survey research books.

Relationships between Variables

One question frequently asked in nursing QA studies is whether or not there is a relationship between two variables of interest. Is there a relationship between patients' anxiety and patients' knowledge of their illness/treatment regimen? Is there a relationship between patient age and length of stay for patients receiving a hip joint replacement? In order to answer such questions, the data on the two variables of interest must be paired by patient so that for each patient the link can be made between the anxiety score and the knowledge score or between the person's age and the number of days spent in the hospital. Relationships between variables such as these, where the measurements are at least approximately at the equal interval level, can be expressed by calculating the Pearson Product Moment Correlation Coefficient, symbolized by r. The Pearson r is an index number that ranges from -1.00 to $+1.00$ and expresses both the direction (indicated by the algebraic sign) and the magnitude (indicated by the absolute value—meaning the size of the index number, regardless of whether it is positive or negative) of the linear relationship between two variables. Absolute values less than .40 are generally described as indicating a weak linear relationship; values in the .40s, .50s, and .60s are moderate; and correlations in the .70s, .80s, and .90s are indications of stronger linear relationships. Perfect correlations of either -1.00 or $+1.00$ are unlikely to be encountered in clinical practice. A value of zero indicates that there is no linear relationship between the two variables.

Because the correlation values themselves are not an equal-interval decimal scale, it is not appropriate to make statements such as an r of .80 is twice the magnitude of an r of .40 or that $r = -.50$ indicates the strength of the relationship is halfway between no relationship and a perfect negative correlation. A simple way to interpret the magnitude of the linear relationship is to square the correlation coefficient to produce r^2, which is called the coefficient of determination. This squared correlation indicates the percentage of variation that is shared by the two variables. If patient age and length of stay are correlated so that $r = .71$, $r^2 = .50$, meaning that knowing a patient's age provides 50 percent of the information needed to predict the patient's length of stay. Conversely, knowing a patient's length of stay provides half the information necessary to predict the patient's age.

The ability to predict from either variable to the other illustrates the fact that a correlation coefficient indicates the degree of association between two variables, but it does not indicate that there is a cause-and-effect relationship. Determining whether or not there is a causal relationship is a question of logic that cannot be answered merely by calculating a correlation coefficient. The fact that squared correlations are always positive numbers serves as a reminder that positive and negative correlations of the same absolute value indicate the same degree of relationship.

The information that is provided by the algebraic sign of a correlation coefficient is the direction of the relationship. A positive sign, which is frequently omitted in writing, indicates that there is a positive or direct relationship where the scores on both variables change in the same direction. A negative sign indicates that there is a negative or inverse relationship where the scores on both variables change in opposite directions. For example, if patient age and length of stay are positively correlated so that $r = .68$, this means that as patient age increases, so does length of stay. If patient age and length of stay are negatively correlated so that $r = -.68$, then as age increases, length of stay decreases. The first correlation allows one to predict that an older patient will have a longer stay than a younger patient, while the second correlation supports the opposite prediction.

It is important to remember that a correlation, like other statistics, refers to the sample on which it is based considered as a group. Except for the atypical case of a perfect correlation where r equals either $+1.00$ or -1.00 so that $r^2 = 1.00$ or 100 percent, it is not true that every older patient will have a longer stay (if r is positive) or shorter stay (if r is negative) than a younger patient. This is simply another example of the same concept illustrated by the fact that not all members of a sample are the same age as the group's mean age except for the atypical case where everyone is the exact same age so that the standard deviation is equal to zero.

Previously, it was noted that a Pearson correlation coefficient equal to zero means that there is no linear relationship between the two variables. This is not the same as saying that there is no relationship of any type between the variables because the Pearson r is designed to determine the existence of relationships that can be described by a straight line. These are the relationships in which people are most frequently interested because they are the easiest to understand and to utilize in practice. When r is zero or some low absolute value, a simple way to determine whether the correlation is low because there is no relationship at all between the variables or because there is only a nonlinear relationship (such as a curvilinear relationship) between the variables is to graph the data to produce what is called a *scatterplot* or *scatter diagram*. Just as with other graphs, one variable such as age is placed on the vertical axis, and the other variable such as length of stay is placed on the horizontal axis. For each patient, a mark is recorded on the graph at the intersection of that patient's age and length of stay values. Examination of the points plotted on the scatter diagram will show either the shape of the nonlinear relationship or no relationship at all, in which case the points will typically fall in a circular pattern.

In addition to its common use as a descriptive statistic, the Pearson correlation is used as an inferential statistic. In this situation, the correlation coefficient calculated from the sample data is used to make an inference about the relationship between the two variables in the population from which the sample was selected. Given that the sample statistic is a correlation value other than zero, the question being asked is whether this is simply due to sampling error (because even carefully selected random samples are not perfectly accurate representations of the population) or whether the population correlation really is different from zero. This question is answered by setting a level of significance (often called the *alpha level*) and performing a test of statistical significance.

For example, if the statement is made that a correlation of $r = .47$ has been calculated for a sample of 32 patients and is significant at the alpha $= .05$ level of significance (which is a very commonly used significance level), this means that there is only a 5 percent chance of being incorrect in inferring that the population correlation is actually different from zero. In other words, if there really is no linear relationship between the two variables in the population, there is only a 5 percent probability that a correlation as large as $r = .47$ would be found to exist in a representative sample drawn from that population. Performing the calculations for this particular example results in the statement that $r = .47$, $p < .01$, meaning that the correlation is statistically significant and that there is less than a 1 percent probability that the population correlation is really zero. Even when a correlation coefficient is statisically significant, it is important to consider the magnitude of the correlation when deciding on the clinical or administrative significance of the relationship represented by the correlation.

Although they are less frequently encountered in the nursing QA literature, there are correlation coefficients other than the Pearson r. The most well known one of these is the Spearman Rank Order Correlation Coefficient, which is symbolized by r_s. As the name implies, the Spearman correlation is used to determine the degree of linear relationship between two ordinal-level variables where the data are reported in terms of ranks. The Spearman r_s has the same possible range of values as the Pearson r and is interpreted in the same manner.

When the nursing QA data of interest are measured at the lowest level of measurement, these nominal-level data can be displayed in a table and analyzed using the Pearson chi-square statistic (symbolized χ^2, using the Greek letter chi) as a test of association to determine if there is a relationship between two variables. With variables measured at the nominal level, such as patient gender, the data are frequencies or counts of how many patients fall into each value or category of the variable—male and female, in this case. If the nursing director of an outpatient clinic concerned with assuring that the clinic is being appropriately staffed for the mix of patients being seen classifies exact patient ages into the three categories of children and adolescents (age 19 or younger), adults (age 20 through 59), and seniors (age 60 or older), this age variable can be cross-tabulated with the gender variable to determine if the two variables are related.

The cross-tabulation or contingency table for this analysis has two dimensions, as shown in Table 10-3, where the three age categories are listed along one dimension and the two gender categories form the other dimension to create a table with six cells. Each cell displays the count of patients who have that particular pair of values; for example, 70 males are older adults. Calculating the chi-square statistic for this contingency table will reveal whether or not there is a statistically significant association between age and gender for this group of 354 patients, but unlike a correlation coefficient, the chi-square cannot provide an indication of the direction and magnitude of the relationship because nominal-level data do not contain that information.

Table 10-3 Number of Patients Using the Ambulatory Care Clinic during July 1990 by Age and Gender

| | Age in Years | | | |
	≤19	20-59	≥60	Totals
Male	37	54	70	161
Female	29	78	86	193
Totals	66	132	156	354

Differences in Patient Care Outcomes

A more common use of chi-square in quality assurance is in assessing outcomes associated with different methods of patient care. For example, as part of a comparison of normal versus heparinized saline for flushing infusion devices, one of the outcomes examined was the number of heparin locks that required restarting because of leaking at the IV site (Taylor, Hutchison, Milliken, & Larson, 1989). Chi-square was used to evaluate the difference in the proportions of leaking locks among the group of patients treated with heparinized saline and the group treated with normal saline. Extrapolating from the reported data to construct a complete cross-tabulation table results in Table 10-4. The chi-square calculated using these data is reported to be statistically significant ($p < .025$), which means that there is less than a 2.5 percent chance of error in stating that there is a difference between the groups. In other words, there is only a small probability that the difference between the 12.9 percent of locks with leaks in the heparin group and the 7.5 percent leaking in the normal saline group is due to chance rather than being a real difference.

Contingency tables are often described in terms of the number of categories there are for the two dimensions (there can actually be more than two dimensions or variables, but the two-variable case is the most commonly encountered situation). Table 10-3 has three categories for the age variable and two values for the gender variable, so it is referred to as a three-by-two table, while Table 10-2 is a two-by-two table. One of the reasons why chi-square is so frequently employed is that it can be used with cross-tabulation tables of many different sizes.

When the clinical or administrative outcomes of interest are measured using instruments that provide basically interval-level data, analyses can be performed

---

Table 10-4 Number of Leaking Intravenous Infusion Devices in the Normal and Heparinized Saline Patient Groups

| | Saline Solution | | |
	Normal	Heparinized	Totals
Leaking	28	46	74
Not leaking	341	310	651
Totals	369	356	725

$\chi^2 = 5.1$, d.f. $= 1$, $p < .025$

Source: Adapted from "Comparison of Normal versus Heparinized Saline for Flushing Infusion Devices" by N. Taylor, E. Hutchison, W. Milliken, and E. Larson, 1989, *Journal of Nursing Quality Assurance*, 3(4), p. 53. Copyright © 1989 by Aspen Publishers, Inc.

to assess the difference in outcome means for two or more comparison groups. An additional outcome examined in the heparin lock study was the length of time it took to flush the infusion device. If the number of seconds it took the nurse to flush the lock was recorded each time the procedure was performed, then the mean number of seconds and the standard deviation could be calculated separately for both the heparin group and the normal saline group.

The difference between these two means can be analyzed by performing a t test, where a t statistic is calculated and tested to determine if it is statistically significant at a specified probability or alpha level, such as .05 or .01. The question being asked of the data is whether the observed difference between the means indicates that the groups really are different in terms of this outcome variable or whether an observed difference of this magnitude is likely to occur simply as a result of chance. If the mean for the heparin group were 140 seconds with a standard deviation of 10 seconds and the comparable statistics for the normal saline group were $M = 87$ seconds and $s = 6$ seconds, the calculated t statistic for groups of the size used in this study would be determined to be statistically significant at $p < .01$. Based on such an analysis, it is reasonable to state (1) that the two groups are significantly different from each other in terms of the average amount of time required to flush the lock and (2) that the probability that this statement is incorrect, such that there really is no difference between the groups, is less than 1 percent.

The t test of a difference between means is only appropriate for comparing two groups. When the means of three or more groups are to be compared, an analysis of variance (ANOVA) procedure is used, which is conceptually an extension of the t test to situations involving more than two groups. In the heparin lock study being used as an example, the heparin group was treated using 10 units/mL heparinized saline. If the study were expanded to include a third group of patients treated using 20 units/mL heparinized saline, the data would be analyzed using an ANOVA procedure where an F test is performed to determine if the calculated F statistic or ratio is statistically significant at the chosen probability level. A determination that the F ratio is statistically significant indicates that the means for the three groups on the outcome variable of time to flush the lock are not all the same. A significant F statistic does not specify which pairs of means are different; it merely reveals that not all the means are equal. In order to determine which pairs of means are different, additional statistical procedures must be performed.

Analysis of variance procedures can also be used for QA studies that simultaneously examine the impact of multiple treatment or organismic variables on an outcome of interest. For example, the heparin study could be extended to determine the outcome differences resulting from type of flushing solution, gauge of catheter, and medical diagnosis that are due to each of these three variables either by themselves or in interaction with one another. When the outcome data of interest are ordinal-level measurements, procedures such as the Kruskal-Wallis and Friedman tests, which are analogous to ANOVA procedures, are available for analyzing the data.

When correlation coefficients were discussed, it was noted that their values fall in the range from -1.00 to $+1.00$ and that the squared coefficient indicates the magnitude of the association. It is not possible to make similar statements for such statistics as chi-square, t, and F. The values of these three statistics are interpreted primarily in terms of statistical significance which is, for a given value of the statistic, dependent on both the alpha probability level chosen and the size of the data set being analyzed. This is also true of correlation coefficients when determining whether or not they are significantly different from zero.

SAMPLE SIZE

The importance of the size of the data set being analyzed has previously been mentioned in several contexts, but a review of some of the issues is worthwhile. A number of cautions should be kept in mind when considering the meaning of statistics calculated for small samples. When percentages are calculated, the size of the group on which they are based still needs to be considered. A 100 percent increase in patient falls on a clinical unit sounds terrible, but may not represent a major threat to patient safety if the number of falls has increased from one to two. The mean and standard deviation of a small group can be quite volatile, even when only one of the scores on which they are based changes in value. This must be considered when using these as descriptive statistics or as part of the calculation of t and F tests. The desirability of comparing means with equivalent stability is one reason why it is recommended that comparison groups be equal in size, especially when the groups are small.

When a sample is randomly selected to represent the larger population of which it is part, the amount of sampling error is directly related to the size of the sample. Larger probability samples represent their population with more precision than do smaller samples selected using the same procedures. This is not necessarily true with nonprobability samples because if there is some systematic bias in how members of the population are selected for the sample, then increasing the sample size may simply compound the amount of error. When it is cost effective to study the entire population (i.e., to conduct a census), there is no sampling error.

A number of methods can be used to decide on an appropriate sample size for a nursing QA study. If the emphasis is on generalizing from the sample to the population, such as when surveys are conducted, one needs to consider how homogeneous the population is, how the data are to be partitioned for analysis, and the types of decisions that will be made based on the data. More heterogeneous populations require larger samples to accurately represent all the variability that exists among the members of the population. Data analysis that will divide the sample into subgroups for comparison requires larger samples to accurately represent the subgroups. Decision making where the consequences of being wrong are severe requires larger samples with less sampling error. Knowing how homogeneous the population is and how much precision is required of the data permits the use of formulas for calculating an appropriate sample size for the study.

If the emphasis is on comparing the impact of differences in clinical or administrative practice, such as when clinical trials or other experiments or quasi-experiments are conducted, one needs to consider the amount of outcome difference it is important to be able to detect. Large outcome differences between groups are easier to detect as being statistically significant while smaller differences are more difficult to detect and so require studies with larger comparison groups that have greater statistical power. Power is basically the ability to detect true outcome differences that exist. Power analysis using the appropriate formulas or tables allows one to choose a sample size that will be neither so small that clinically meaningful differences are overlooked nor so large that meaningless differences are statistically significant. Statistical significance is a good screening mechanism in that it provides a statement of the probability that the observed results are simply due to chance, but it is not an assurance of clinical or practical significance, which is a much different judgment that needs to be made. Guidance for determining a reasonable sample size for a particular QA study can be found in research textbooks and in specialized volumes on the topic, such as that of Kramer and Thiemann (1987).

DATA AND NURSING QA DECISIONS

In order to make sound clinical and administrative decisions that will help assure the provision of quality patient care, it is necessary to have accurate information that has been effectively analyzed to provide a basis for such decisions. Statistics can be a powerful tool for facilitating this decision-making process, provided that the appropriate variables have been reliably and validly measured. Statistical formulas are not magic incantations capable of turning meaningless numbers into useful data. What statistics can do is to organize data into meaningful configurations that can be readily understood and communicated.

Taking a cue from the fields of architecture and design, sometimes less really is more when it comes to making an impact. Providing people with a large number of individual measurements quickly becomes overwhelming. Summarizing the information about each variable of interest and showing how the variables interrelate through the use of tables, graphs, and statistics focuses attention on the meaning of the data and makes for a much more effective presentation.

An important use of nursing QA data is to provide feedback to staff to help guide their actions. This feedback is most useful to people when it is put into some sort of comparative context, such as by showing the current level of an indicator variable compared to the level during prior time periods and/or to the established criterion level. Figure 10-1 is an example of such a comparison. In a similar fashion, the impact of a care procedure on patient outcomes is most easily evaluated in comparison to alternative care procedures also aimed at influencing those same outcomes. This is why well-designed clinical trials always include comparison groups of patients receiving different care protocols. Table 10-4 is an example of this type of comparison.

The informed application of even basic statistical procedures greatly facilitates QA decision making and explicates the rationale for the decisions so that they can be readily understood by others. This places one in a much stronger position for gaining genuine support for and knowledgeable compliance with the recommended course of action. The application of statistics to health care data has been important to nursing quality assurance since Florence Nightingale pioneered the approach, and it has never been more necessary and important than it is in the current increasingly complex health care environment.

REFERENCES

Barget, C.D., & Zink, M.R. (1989). Evaluation of clinical indicators in IV home care. *Journal of Nursing Quality Assurance, 3*(3), 64–74.

Hays, W.L. (1988). *Statistics* (4th ed.). New York: Holt, Rinehart & Winston.

Jaffe, A.J., & Spirer, H.F. (1987). *Misused statistics: Straight talk for twisted numbers.* New York: Marcel Dekker.

Knapp, R.G. (1985). *Basic statistics for nurses* (2nd ed.). New York: Wiley.

Kramer, H.C., & Thiemann, S. (1987). *How many subjects? Statistical power analysis in research.* Newbury Park, CA: Sage.

Robertson, M.M., & DeCampli, P.D. (1988). Infection control rounds: A method for evaluating safety. *Journal of Nursing Quality Assurance, 3*(1), 46–56.

Taylor, N., Hutchison, E., Milliken, W., & Larson, E. (1989). Comparison of normal versus heparinized saline for flushing infusion devices. *Journal of Nursing Quality Assurance, 3*(4), 49–55.

Volicer, B.J. (1984). *Multivariate statistics for nursing research.* Orlando: Grune & Stratton.

Waltz, C.F., Strickland, O.L., & Lenz, E.R. (1984). *Measurement in nursing research.* Philadelphia: F.A. Davis.

11

Clinical Interpretation and Analysis of Monitoring Data

Marie J. Driever, PhD, RN, Assistant Director of Nursing, Quality Assurance/Research, Providence Medical Center, Portland, Oregon

INTRODUCTION AND PURPOSE

The goal of quality assurance (QA) is the improvement of patient care. The challenge of implementing a meaningful and relevant QA plan is twofold: to demonstrate that quality assurance leads to improved patient care and to increase the skill of staff in a component of the QA process so that improvement can and will occur. The purposes of this chapter are to

- define the QA process component of interpretation
- explain the premises and principles of interpretation as applied to the QA process
- distinguish methods, analysis, and interpretation in terms of their distinct features
- outline a procedure for interpreting QA data
- describe an environment in which interpretation will provide direction for improved patient care and strengthen the practice of nursing

DEFINITION OF TERMS

Smeltzer, Hinshaw, and Feltman (1987) have defined nursing quality assurance with a focus that is helpful in understanding the component of interpretation. Nursing quality assurance is the "systematic testing or evaluation of nursing practice" (Smeltzer, Hinshaw, & Feltman, 1987, p. 2). This definition highlights the concept of systematic testing. In other words, quality assurance is a continuous and interactive process with judgments made at strategic points about the aspects of care being monitored *and* the process itself. Evaluation is at the core of this

239

interactive process. Data generated from ongoing monitoring and evaluation enable nurses to determine what changes are needed in nursing practice in order to improve patient care (Smeltzer, Hinshaw, & Feltman, 1987).

Currently the Joint Commission on Accreditation of Healthcare Organizations has a ten-step monitoring and evaluation process it describes as the cornerstone of effective QA activities (Joint Commission on Accreditation of Healthcare Organizations, 1988). Interpretation is integral to several of the Joint Commission's ten steps.

- Step 6: Collect and organize data.
- Step 7: Evaluate care.
- Step 8: Take actions to solve problems.
- Step 9: Assess actions and document improvement. (Joint Commission, 1988, pp. 50–57).

The Joint Commission describes the QA program as "one essential component of efforts to ensure continuous improvement in the quality of patient care" (Joint Commission, 1988, p. 45). The cognitive and interactive process of interpretation provides the means and momentum for the ongoing evaluation required for continuous quality improvement.

For the purposes of this chapter, interpretation, based on the work of Kerlinger (1986), is defined as explaining or finding meaning. As with the research process, QA findings "are not meaningful until they are interpreted" (Burns & Grove, 1987, p. 59). To continue borrowing from the research process, findings generated by QA activities are examined for their credibility in the context of how the monitoring was conceptualized, planned, and actually carried out (Woods & Catanzaro, 1988, p. 11).

Interpretation consists of taking the summarized data, examining these data for patterns, describing these patterns, drawing conclusions, and determining implications for changes to improve patient care. These aspects of interpretation provide the basis for comparing the fit between the performance indicated by the data and the predetermined threshold indicating the required level of accomplishment (Driever, 1988, p. 56). This ongoing comparison of the fit between the level of quality to be achieved and the meaning attributed to the results of monitoring helps nurses to know if care is being improved. In this way interpretation as a critical component of the QA process stimulates continuous quality improvement.

PREMISES AND PRINCIPLES OF INTERPRETATION IN THE QA PROCESS

Interpretation involves a search for the meaning and implications of the findings obtained from monitoring activities. Identification of implications relates to two aspects of change. One is determining appropriate corrective action and/or opportunities for care improvement. The second is determining the effectiveness of the QA plan in promoting relevant monitoring whereby evaluation against preestablished standards of practice excellence will occur.

Findings are examined for their meaning in relation to the individual indicator, the purposes for monitoring the indicator, the identified clinical functions, the data collection plan, the data elements used to operationalize the indicator, and the predetermined threshold. Based on this examination, interpretation of findings leads to the drawing of inferences pertinent to conclusions about the QA data.

Interpretation requires cognitive activity by individual nurses, followed by discussion of the findings and identification of the implications by a community of nurse peers. Given the unit-based focus of QA activities (Schroeder & Maibusch, 1984), the community of nurse peers initially needs to be the staff nurses who practice on the unit. Monitoring activities provide each unit's community of peers with the bases for evaluating the care they provide both on a daily basis and over time for their high-volume, high-risk, and special problem patient populations. In addition to unit-level peers, there is merit in structuring opportunities for both nurse managers and staff nurses across units to share their interpretations of unit-based QA results. Through such ongoing discussion of findings, and, more importantly, through the interpretation of those findings, all levels of nurses from staff through administration can identify trends and issues relating to the level of care provided patients and can develop and then monitor strategies to improve trends and resolve issues of concern.

METHODS, ANALYSIS, AND INTERPRETATION

The terms *methods, analysis*, and *interpretation* connote the research process. Indeed, it is a major thesis of this chapter that aspects of the research process can inform, thereby providing direction and a basis for strengthening the QA process. The concepts of methods, analysis, and interpretation are described using characteristics from the research process to further develop these concepts for the QA process.

Methods refer to the general strategy and procedures planned to accomplish monitoring of each indicator. The concept of measurement is critical in considering the strategy by which monitoring will occur. Measurement is "the process of assigning numbers to objects, events or situations in accord with some rule" (Burns & Grove, 1987, p. 748). The data elements developed to operationalize each indicator must be specific and sufficiently circumscribed for assignment of a numbering system.

Most often the numbering system used for the monitoring process reflects the presence or absence of a desired care aspect. This presence or absence of each data element must be translated into items on a data collection sheet; for example, a

"1" may be assigned to indicate presence, and "0," absence. In this instance the rule for numbering is to determine whether the presence or absence is to be consistently counted in assessing whether compliance with the threshold was achieved. Thus, if the indicator focus is the performance of identified patient teaching behaviors, the data collection items must be worded so the scores consist of points assigned for items that are present; these point values can then be added to obtain a total score that can be compared with the indicator threshold. In this example the presence of patient teaching behaviors or the consistency with which patient teaching behaviors were performed would be a basis for measuring this indicator.

In deciding the measurement approach it is critical to have congruence among the following elements: (1) the focus of the indicator, (2) the purpose for monitoring, (3) the data elements identified to operationalize the indicator, and (4) the approach or strategy to collect data. Most often, the general strategy consists of a chart review approach, either concurrent or retrospective, to data collection. In designing methods for quality assurance, research and evaluation principles related to instrument development, use of a variety of ways to collect data (e.g., observation, survey, and interview), and consideration of the reliability and validity of the measures should be applied as much as is appropriate and relevant (Bloch, 1975, 1980).

Answering certain questions provides guidance for decision makers who must determine the methods for each indicator. What will be measured? How often? By what method, and by whom? How many patients will serve as subjects? (Coyne & Killien, 1987). The first question—What will be measured?—is a priority and must be answered early in the design of methods because the answer to this question provides direction for developing the procedural aspects of QA methods. The object of measurement relates to operationalizing the concepts and/or dimensions of each identified indicator so that relevant data will be obtained from data collection activities. For example, for an indicator such as "Planning is individualized for each patient," critical concepts to operationalize are "planning" and "individualized." The standards of care dictated by hospital policies and/or desired practice within the nursing community can help to determine the data elements to measure and the level of value that indicates desired and acceptable performance.

Delineation of the data elements required to measure an indicator provides the basis for a data collection form. Again using as a sample indicator the individualized plan of care for each patient, the data elements that are selected to operationalize relevant standards and that serve as data collection items are (1) assessment completed within eight hours of patient admission and (2) care plan includes specific behavioral goals for patient.

While quality assurance is most often associated with a chart review approach, other ways to collect data that may more precisely measure the indicator should be considered. These include paper/pencil surveys, observations, and interviews. It is critical to expand consideration of data collection methods beyond chart review. As the focus of quality measurement moves to one of patient outcomes achieved, it will be necessary to use a variety of methods. The kinds of methods used have implications for interpretation of the QA data. The major implication relates to the level of development of the instrument used to collect data. For example, chart review forms are usually developed as an indicator is identified. The data collection sheets then need to be critically reviewed to see that the forms have sufficient items to operationalize all relevant facets of quality to be measured by the indicator. The stage of development (i.e., whether initial development or a revision based on previous use) needs to be taken into account during analysis and interpretation of results.

In addition to determining the design and measurement strategy, the other methods components consist of descriptions of the data collection procedures, the sample to be obtained, and the ways in which the data will be analyzed. The description of the data collection procedures includes who will collect the data, how the data will be collected, and how compliance will be determined. For example, staff nurse Ann Jones will do concurrent chart review of all charts of all patients with a two-day postoperative status on every Wednesday of the quarter. It is anticipated that 10 patient charts will be reviewed every week, for a total of 120 per quarter, which is 25 percent of the population of postoperative patients. Compliance will be determined by counting the presence of each data collection item, adding the scores, and comparing the total score with the identified indicator threshold.

Analysis refers to the procedures used to categorize, organize, and summarize the data to produce findings that must then be interpreted (Burns & Grove, 1987; Kerlinger, 1986). According to Fitz-Gibbon and Morris (1987), the first step in data analysis is to examine the score for each item on the data collection instrument and then to determine a way of ordering the scores as a basis for summarizing them. Most often analysis involves the use of quantitative procedures such as adding and averaging responses to items from the data collection instruments. This summation, which yields a percentage score that indicates how often the data items occurred, is referred to as the level of compliance. The level of compliance is then compared to the threshold set for each indicator. The most fundamental and most common analysis procedure determines compliance by means of comparing actual scores with the set threshold. After the total score is obtained, it is then helpful to examine the data by item and by groups of items. Such an examination provides for the identification of trends, both positive and negative. These trends can be described in terms of what desired aspects of compliance are high, and possibly which of these could still be improved, whereas desired aspects that are low in compliance point to areas where corrective action should be taken. If analysis stops there, however, potential meanings of the data will be overlooked.

Methods and analyses set the stage for the critical component of the QA process: interpretation (Driever, 1988).

Interpretation, as previously defined, is the assignment of meaning to data. As such, interpretation requires methods of data collection that will allow sufficient and relevant data to be obtained and analysis that will organize the data so interpretations can be made. Interpretation is the pulling together of the data so that implications and recommendations can be delineated and implemented as a basis for improving patient care.

INTERPRETING QA DATA

Several procedures are required in order to interpret QA data. Interpretation involves (1) summarizing the data, (2) analyzing or examining issues of measurement, (3) analyzing or identifying trends in the data, and (4) developing conclusions and determining implications and recommended actions.

Summarizing the Data

The purpose of summarizing is to consolidate and present the data collected for each indicator and to prepare them for analysis. Summarizing the data involves collating and organizing the data by item from the data collection sheet. A data summary sheet is highly recommended in order to handle data easily and efficiently (King, Morris, & Fitz-Gibbon, 1987). In most instances data are summarized for manual analysis. However, for large amounts of data or for more extensive analysis, it is advisable to use a computer with appropriate statistical software. For this kind of analysis, resources on what statistical tests to use, as well as on how to use the software to perform the statistical procedure, should be consulted. A data sheet, however, is usable for both manual and computer analysis. Exhibit 11-1 contains an example of a data sheet. Such data summary sheets help with data interpretation because they assist in identifying patterns of response (King, Morris, & Fitz-Gibbon, 1987). The patterns of response identified provide the basis for attributing meaning and identifying implications.

Since manual scoring is still the most frequent mode of analysis for QA data, the use of a quick-tally sheet will be described as an example of how to use a data sheet. A quick-tally sheet displays all response options for each item so you can tally the number of times people chose an item or the number of times an item referred to was present/absent in the patient care record (King, Morris, & Fitz-Gibbon, 1987, p. 115). A data summary sheet requires either closed-response data or open-ended responses that have been categorized and coded. Closed-response data include results from structured observation instruments, interviews,

Exhibit 11-1 Data Sheet

INDICATOR: Are patients' glucose levels assessed appropriately, and is necessary follow-up initiated?

Threshold: 96%

Items on Data Collection Sheet	Possible Responses	Yes	No	NA	% Compliance (Yes) Responses
a. Patient's blood glucose level is monitored according to physician/nurse schedule (+1 − 30")	294	257	37	—	87
b. Orders are present to administer sliding scale insulin (or oral agent) and/or to notify MD	294	273	21	—	93
c. Nurse administered correct amount of insulin (or oral agent) or called physician as required for appropriate follow-up response.*	294	119	27	148	91

Overall Compliance 90%

*Because follow-up action based on level of patient's blood glucose may not always be necessary, compliance response is computed by adding the number of "yes" and "NA" responses.

Source: Adapted with permission of Providence Medical Center Nursing Staff, Surgical Unit, Portland, OR.

questionnaires, and chart audit forms, which produce tallies or numbers (King, Morris, & Fitz-Gibbon, 1987, p. 115). Tallies for QA data most often are in the form of yes/no or present/absent responses. However, the response set can take the Likert format with 0–9 as possible scores. This series of interval responses reflects asking a degree response (e.g., how much agreement/disagreement some people believe exists) as their response to the focus of each item on the questionnaire.

Careful construction of the data sheet will provide for the analysis of all relevant data. The data collection sheet must contain all the items for each criterion used to operationalize the indicator. Using Exhibit 11-1 as an example, the three items listed reflect the criterion of blood sugar monitoring according to physician/nurse schedule as the operational definition of the portion of the indicator relating to whether patients' glucose levels were assessed appropriately. A quick-tally sheet allows calculation of two possible descriptive statistics: (1) the number and percentage of each possible response to each item (e.g., the number of yes/present responses) and/or (2) the average response to each item (with standard deviation) in cases where an average is a meaningful summary (e.g., where the response set is a degree such as 0, 1, 2, 3) (King, Morris & Fitz-Gibbon, 1987, p. 115). The quick-tally sheet allows summarization of how many or what percentage of the group responded in a particular way to each item and to all the items as a whole (King, Morris, & Fitz-Gibbon, 1987, p. 116).

However, in addition to the major indicator data element items, gathering data on related elements may be beneficial. These related data elements pertain to specific shifts, units, age, sex, and/or diagnosis of patients. Thus, these related elements need to be included in the construction of the data collection sheet and then included in the data display sheet.

If there is interest in making more detailed analyses, such as correlating the response patterns of individuals within the data sample, use of a computer is advisable in order to do this most efficiently. If, however, a manual method of analysis is preferred or required, a second kind of data sheet, the people-item data roster, will be useful. On this kind of roster, the data collection items are listed across the top of the page. The people, shift, and other related data elements are listed in a vertical column on the left. These elements are usually identified by number so as to allow large amounts of data to be summarized on one sheet. Graph paper or the kind of paper used for computer programming is useful for constructing these data rosters, even when the data are to be processed by hand rather than by computer (King, Morris, & Fitz-Gibbon, 1987, p. 116). Exhibit 11-2 shows how Exhibit 11-1 can be revised to include one kind of related data element, nurse shifts.

Analysis As Examination for Issues of Measurement

The purpose of this aspect of the procedure is to review the design strategy, the data collection instruments and procedures used to measure the indicator, and the

Exhibit 11-2 Data Sheet with Related Element of Data by Shift

INDICATOR: Are patients' glucose levels assessed appropriately, and is necessary follow-up initiated?

Threshold: 96%

Items on Data Collection Sheet	Possible Responses	Yes	No	NA	% Compliance (Yes) Responses
a. Patient's blood glucose level is monitored according to physician/nurse schedule (+1 − 30″)	294	257	37	—	87
b. Data by shift*	257				
Days		200	17	—	78
Eves		47	16	—	18
Nocs		10	4	—	4
c. Orders are present to administer sliding scale insulin (or oral agent) and/or to notify MD	294	273	5	80	97
d. Nurse administered correct amount of insulin (or oral agent) or called physician as required for appropriate follow-up response.**	294	119	27	148	91

Overall Compliance 90%

*To compute compliance responses for data element by shift, number of "yes" responses is used as the denominator.
**Because follow-up action based on level of patient's blood glucose may not always be necessary, compliance response is computed by adding the number of "yes" and "NA" responses.

Source: Adapted with permission of Providence Medical Center Nursing Staff, Surgical Unit, Portland, OR.

systematic nature of the data collection. The data, which have been summarized as outlined earlier in this interpretation procedure, provide the basis for reviewing how well each indicator was measured. To do this, certain questions need to be asked: Are the data complete? What else could have been measured to help determine the level of quality reflected by the indicator? In this way, whether there are sufficient data elements to operationalize the indicator and whether these elements are clearly stated so data collectors can consistently collect the required data are evaluated. Based on this examination, the data collection sheets may be revised by expanding the number of items and/or clarifying the statement of the items. In addition, sampling procedures and data collection procedures may be revised to simplify and strengthen data collection. If data collection instruments are appropriate, internal consistency reliability testing needs to be done and the results used to evaluate the strength of the measurement for each indicator. In this way the QA process of design and data collection will be improved and will assure that sufficient and relevant data are consistently obtained.

Analysis As Identification of Trends in the Data

The purpose here is to provide complete analyses of the data. The initial aspect of data analysis is to examine the scores for each item and try to describe the results conveyed by the data. This item-by-item review and then the overall review of the data provide a look at what the scores are and then at what picture emerges from the data. In the example in Exhibit 11-1 the picture that emerges is one of compliance with two items reflecting two indicator data elements. However, one item score is below the determined indicator threshold. There is also a pattern of response according to the shifts nurses work.

This examination of the findings in terms of data collection items is the start of analyzing the data in relation to the indicator. The examination is completed by asking these questions: Do the data fit the indicator? If yes, how well? If no, what aspects are missing? The goal is to judge how well the data fit the focus of the indicator. A sample indicator with the focus on the patient outcome of "satisfaction with care" provides clarification. The data on patient satisfaction were collected using the Hinshaw and Atwood Survey of Patient Satisfaction (Hinshaw & Atwood, 1982). The data obtained from this instrument yield three scores (one for each subscale of the instrument): technical-professional care, trust, and patient education. A total satisfaction score is also calculated. To determine if the data fit this indicator, each subscale score must be examined to assess whether it reflects patient satisfaction. How well this measure operationalized patient satisfaction was determined as part of deciding how the data were to be collected during the QA plan design phase. However, during the analysis phase, examination of data scores focuses on the fit between the indicator and the data and provides the bases for determining whether the data sufficiently answer the indicator and whether additional or different aspects are needed. The instrument used in the patient satisfaction survey example has items relating to the timeliness of care provided. Perhaps there need to be more of these items or items relating to the staff's timely response to the patient's family as well. This step ends with a description of the patterns within the data collected. Patterns of compliance and noncompliance with indicator criteria need to be identified and described in a narrative. Such examination and description provide a basis for a broader focus—explaining and seeking meaning.

Developing Conclusions and Determining Implications and Recommended Actions

The purposes of this aspect of the procedure are to describe (1) what the data mean, (2) what inferences can be drawn from the data, and (3) what possible implications for the level of care quality can be identified. The study results are compared to the standards for each indicator and possibly to other people's findings as well (Driever, 1988; Kerlinger, 1986). To complete this step, the narrative describing the quantitative data must be added. This narrative should be developed in a stepwise fashion, starting with a description of the findings for each item and/or each subscale. The next step is to highlight the trends in the data by groupings of items, by subscale, and/or in relation to nurse performance characteristics (unit, shift) and/or patient characteristics (age, gender, diagnosis). The description of trends, patterns, and themes in the data is basic to interpretation. These trends are described as to their highs and lows in relation to the indicator threshold. Based on this description, conclusions are then drawn as to what these trends, patterns, and themes mean in terms of the level of care quality, and why and how these patterns are occurring. The conclusions drawn from the description (i.e., what the results are and what they mean) provide the explanation and, therefore, the rationale for recommended actions. These recommended actions may be corrective in nature if the data indicate compliance below the set indicator threshold, or they may provide opportunities for quality improvement if compliance matches or exceeds the indicator threshold.

According to Pinkerton (1988, p. 52), critical thinking is "a process of defining and analyzing problems, with the emphasis on questioning information rather than merely accepting it." In the current complex care environment, nurses need this skill in "reviewing physicians' orders, incorporating standard policies and procedures in practice, reviewing accepted nursing interventions and interpreting patient data" (Pinkerton, 1988, p. 52). The procedure for the interpretation of data outlines how to accomplish this component of the QA process. The discussion of this procedure also highlights the integrated nature of the QA process. Being integral to quality assurance as a monitoring and evaluation process, interpretation is dependent on what is selected to be measured as indicators of quality and on the strategies and procedures selected for measurement as the bases for making judgments. Making judgments or determining meaning serves as the impetus for staff response to "findings made visible through which improvement in quality occurs" (Coyne & Killien, 1987, p. 77). Interpretation provides the means for understanding the results obtained from monitoring activities and for refining the QA plan in order to strengthen the process of evaluating care delivery.

AN ENVIRONMENT THAT NURTURES INTERPRETATION

The clinical analysis and interpretation of monitoring data require a systematic process of evaluation. For this process to be relevant, a certain kind of environment is required. This environment is one that nurtures all components of the QA process, but most especially that of interpretation. The descriptor of nurturing was selected to convey the required support and promotion of the skills, competence, and motivation for continual improvement of quality care and the process to evaluate it.

Two conditions must be in place for a nurturing environment to exist. One condition relates to the beliefs held by the staff: that quality assurance assures quality of care and that those involved in quality assurance promote change (Bliersbach, 1988, p. 318). A related belief is that staff involved in quality assurance have a role and actively work on developing QA data elements based on "group judgment methods" (Williamson, 1971). Group judgment is supported through the peer relationship process (Gerstner, McAllister, Wagner, & Kraus, 1988), the second condition for an environment that nurtures the QA process.

Being a member of a nursing unit provides the opportunity for all the nurses not only to care cooperatively for patients, but also, more importantly, to form a community of professional peers. One result of a unit-based QA program is the creation of a designated community of peers. Professional peers relate to each other to exchange knowledge, aid, support, and evaluative feedback as a basis for evaluating and strengthening their practice of nursing. A unit-based nursing staff that practices nursing as a community of peers is able to challenge the members as individuals and as a group of professionals toward more critical thinking about their own and their peers' practice.

Acting as a community of peers, nursing unit staff have a critical stake in assuring an excellent level of practice for their patient populations. As such, the members of each nursing unit's nursing staff then become stakeholders. Stakeholders are people who have a "stake, a vested interest in evaluation findings" (Patton, 1987, p. 43). Stakeholders make decisions and use information obtained from monitoring and evaluation activities. Because of the vested interests of stakeholders, the QA plan must be developed to incorporate their questions, needs, and issues so that stakeholders will use evaluation information (Guba & Lincoln, 1989).

Being a stakeholder and an interpreter of QA data in order to improve the day-to-day practice of nursing requires an interactive process. Each nurse must identify and communicate individually valued aspects of care to serve as the bases for QA activities. Then the nurse community of peers must work to meld individually valued aspects into data elements for the community's QA program, thereby determining each unit's image of what constitutes excellent practice.

The data obtained by QA activities are translated into usable information through interpretation. As previously outlined, interpretation is the creation of meaning from QA results. The community of peers creates meaning through individual reviews of the data and peer debriefing. Building on the work of Guba and Lincoln (1989), peer debriefing refers to the process of engaging each other in discussions of findings, analyses, and conclusions, the purpose of which is to test out, and thereby develop the meaning of, QA results. Each individual, acting as a peer, poses searching questions and tentative analyses in order to construct the meaning of QA data and results. Peer debriefing contributes to a process of interaction whereby nurses become systematic testers of their practice. An environment that provides opportunities for such interactions will contribute to answering the question of how to motivate nurses to change their practice (Duquette, 1989).

Monitoring has effectively been described as just the beginning in that QA data are the "stepping stones for actions necessary to improve care" (Mottet, 1987, p. 27). QA monitoring must occur within an environment that nurtures interpretation. Such an environment supports and promotes a process of peer interaction that challenges the testing of nursing practice and that reflects continuous monitoring for care improvement.

REFERENCES

Bliersbach, C.M. (1988). Quality assurance in health care: Current challenges and future directions. *Quality Review Bulletin, 14*(10), 315–319.

Bloch, D. (1975). Evaluation of nursing care in terms of process and outcome: Issues in research and quality assurance. *Nursing Research, 24*(4), 256–263.

Bloch, D. (1980). Interrelated issues in evaluation and evaluation research: A researcher's perspective. *Nursing Research, 20*(2), 69–73.

Burns, N., & Grove, S.K. (1987). *The practice of nursing research: Conduct, critique, and utilization.* Philadelphia: W.B. Saunders.

Coyne, C., & Killien, M. (1987). A system for unit-based monitors of quality of nursing care. *Journal of Nursing Administration, 17*(1), 26–32.

Driever, M.J. (1988). Interpretation: A critical component of the quality assurance process. *Journal of Nursing Quality Assurance, 2*(2), 55–58.

Duquette, A. (1989). Implementing corrective action plans with power. *Journal of Nursing Quality Assurance, 3*(4), 9–14.

Gerstner, M., McAllister, L., Wagner, P.L., & Kraus, C. (1988). Peer review. In S.E. Pinkerton & P. Schroeder (Eds.), *Commitment to excellence* (pp. 199–209). Gaithersburg, MD: Aspen Publishers.

Guba, E.G., & Lincoln, Y.S. (1989). *Fourth generation evaluation.* Newbury Park, CA: Sage.

Hinshaw, A.S., & Atwood, J.R. (1982). A patient satisfaction instrument: Precision by replication. *Nursing Research, 31*(3), 170–191.

Joint Commission on Accreditation of Healthcare Organizations. (1988). *The Joint Commission guide to quality assurance.* Chicago: Author.

Kerlinger, F.N. (1986). Principles of analysis and interpretation. In *Foundations of behavioral research* (3rd ed.). New York: CBS College.

King, J.A., Morris, L.L., & Fitz-Gibbon, C.T. (1987). *How to assess program implementation.* Newbury Park, CA: Sage.

Mottet, E.A. (1987). Monitoring is only the beginning. *Journal of Nursing Quality Assurance, 1*(3), 23–27.

Patton, M.Q. (1987). *Utilization-focused evaluation.* Newbury Park, CA: Sage.

Pinkerton, S.E. (1988). Critical thinking: Integration of a concept. In: S.E. Pinkerton & P. Schroeder (Eds.), *Commitment to excellence* (pp. 51–57). Gaithersburg, MD: Aspen Publishers.

Schroeder, P.S., & Maibusch, R.M. (Eds.). (1984). *Nursing quality assurance: A unit-based approach.* Gaithersburg, MD: Aspen Publishers.

Smeltzer, C.H., Feltman, B., & Rajki, K. (1983). Nursing quality assurance: A process, not a tool. *Journal of Nursing Administration, 13*(1), 5–9.

Smeltzer, C.H., Hinshaw, A.S., & Feltman, B. (1987). The benefits of staff nurse involvement in monitoring the quality of patient care. *Journal of Nursing Quality Assurance, 1*(3), 1–7.

Taylor Fitz-Gibbon, C., & Morris, L.L. (1987). *How to analyze data.* Newbury Park, CA: Sage.

Williamson, J.W. (1971). Evaluating quality of patient care: A strategy relating outcome and process assessment. *Journal of American Medical Association, 218*(4), 564–569.

Woods, N.F. (1988). Interpreting the findings. In N.F. Woods & M. Catanzaro (Eds.), *Nursing research: Theory and practice* (pp. 457–465). St. Louis: C.V. Mosby.

Woods, N.F., & Catanzaro, M. (1988). Generating nursing science. In N.F. Woods & M. Catanzaro (Eds.), *Nursing research: Theory and practice* (pp. 3–17). St. Louis: C.V. Mosby.

12

Changing Practice: An Overview

Angeline Bushy, PhD, RN, *Assistant Professor, College of Nursing Community Health, University of Utah, Salt Lake City, Utah*

INTRODUCTION

Our world is changing so quickly that it has become increasingly difficult to keep up with new developments—much less understand them. Consequently, everyone knows that change is inevitable—if not always welcome. Change is necessary for growth, but it can produce anxiety and fear. Planned or unplanned, change can be threatening because it is the process of making something different than what has been. Even when change is desired, an individual has a sense of loss of the familiar. These feelings are more pronounced when change results from unplanned circumstances, but grief reactions can occur even when change is anticipated.

Problem solving serves as the conceptual structure for the change process, as well as the scientific method, the diagnostic process, the teaching process, the research process, and the nursing process. All of these processes consist of logical, sequential, conscious, and deliberate activities. Change is not unique to any one profession; however, the theory must be tailored for each discipline. Change theory provides a commonality, a universal language, among the disciplines regarding the change process (American Nurses' Association, 1980; Drucker, 1974; Sullivan & Decker, 1988).

This chapter will define frequently used terms associated with change, outline several classic change theories, explore the role of change in quality assurance (QA) activities, and discuss strategies that can be used by quality assurance coordinators (QACs) to fulfill their designated responsibilities.

DEFINITIONS

The following terms and their definitions are used in this chapter.

Change agent refers to a manager of change—that is, one who sets out to bring about a change by utilizing a systematic body of knowledge. In quality assurance, the manager of change usually is a QAC. This individual is often mandated to make changes within a particular setting (system); however, a prior verbal or written mandate from another party is not essential (Havelock, 1973; Lewin, 1951; Lippitt, 1973; Sullivan & Decker, 1988).

For nurses, change is often initiated from within an organization by an associate (insider) who is seeking to make an impact on nursing services (American Nurses' Association, 1980). Likewise, one who is designated as QAC has a significant role in bringing about systemwide changes. But, with quality assurance, staff nurses and others may recognize the need for a change within the hospital. For this reason, staff-level employees may now find the need to initiate changes, a responsibility at one time expected only of managers. Still, to provide consistency in the use of terms in this chapter, *change agent* and *quality assurance coordinator* are used as synonyms.

Changee refers to the group that is being changed within a system (Havelock, 1973; Lewin, 1951; Lippitt, 1973; Sullivan & Decker, 1988). for the QAC, the changee can be a particular individual, a clinical unit, a specific department, an institution, or an entire health care system. Even though staff members may be in a position to initiate change as a part of quality assurance, in this chapter the terms *professionals* and *associates* will be substituted for *changee* for the sake of clarity.

Change refers to that group of activities, as well as of resources (time, money, personnel), required to bring about a modification or to implement a vision (Havelock, 1973; Lewin, 1951; Lippitt, 1973; Sullivan & Decker, 1988).

The term *innovation*, a similar concept, is defined as an object, process, practice, or idea that is totally or partially new to a potential adopter, an institution, or the entire world. Acceptance of an innovation mandates numerous changes on the part of those who adopt it (Drucker, 1985a, 1985b; Rogers, 1971). Hence, the terms *innovation* and *change* will be used interchangeably.

More specifically, within the last decade quality assurance has been an innovation to health care professionals. This has necessitated numerous changes on the part of those who work in these settings. These changes include implementing QA plans, identifying standards of practice, determining indicators, monitoring practice and outcomes, establishing protocols, and following up investigated problems. All of these should ultimately improve the quality of patient care.

Change can be a planned or an unplanned event. *Unplanned change* usually results from a set of random events that brings about one or more unpredictable outcomes. These circumstantial outcomes may be favorable, unfavorable, or a combination of the two (Havelock, 1973; Lewin, 1951; Lippitt, 1973; Sullivan & Decker, 1988).

Planned change, on the other hand, is an orchestrated sequence of events, implemented to achieve a defined goal, outcome, or vision. This process includes determining driving and restraining forces that facilitate or impede achieving a predetermined outcome. To rephrase, some individuals desire change because they anticipate personal or professional gains. Others resist change because they experience anxiety due to the poorly defined expectations and/or the loss of the status quo (Lewin, 1951; Marriner, 1979).

Figure 12-1 depicts the change process in relation to QA activities. The figure correlates terms from change theory with QA terms. Incidentally, *change agent* can be substituted for *quality assurance coordinator; changee* refers to the professionals or associates on a particular unit, department, or institution; *change (innovation)* can be substituted for the term *quality assurance activities*. Finally, *planned change* is another term for *quality assurance outcomes*.

HEALTH CARE: A CLIMATE FOR CHANGE

Toffler (1970), later Naisbitt (1983), and more recently Peters and Austin (1985) depict a global scenario of rapid change. This is partly due to a shift in demographic patterns, increased mobility of the population, accessibility to informatic systems, and availability of complex technology.

Consequently, the modern world demands a reordering of almost everything that we have come to learn, love, and appreciate, and with which we are comfortable. All change, no matter how small, has a rippling effect that impacts numerous other entities (subsystems). These global changes have mandated flexibility as individuals and organizations respond to change. In essence, creative

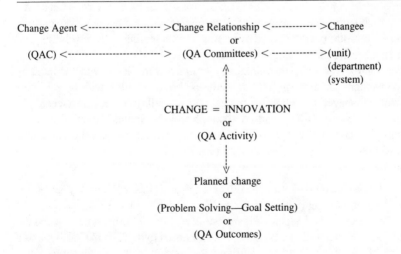

Figure 12-1 Change Process Applied to a QA Program

change has become critical for survival, health, and growth in modern society (Hersey & Blanchard, 1977).

For the business of health care, many changes are economically driven. This is perpetuated by such external forces as the national health policy, third-party payers, and employers who have attempted to alter well-established reimbursement practices that condone a blank-check consumer mentality. Internal and external forces, such as the ones mentioned, have mandated the need for health care institutions to carefully monitor the quality, as well as the cost effectiveness, of their product. Based on these findings, an organization must have the ability to respond rapidly in order to modify its infrastructure, technology, and/or staffing patterns (Rakich, Longest, & O'Donovan, 1977).

CHANGE AND QUALITY ASSURANCE

The question arises, What needs to be changed in health care? Four general categories (situations) are identified.

1. *Dysfunction within an organization.* Examples of this include power struggles between various clinical units, personality conflicts in a particular department, lack of cohesiveness among the employees in carrying out team responsibilities to achieve the hospital's overall goal, and low morale among the employees.
2. *Expansion of the capabilities of an existing organization.* Examples of this include adding new services or departments within a hospital, developing new community educational programs, implementing outreach clinics, and restructuring an existing department.
3. *Recognition of a missing function.* Examples of this include the demand by consumers for new surgical procedures, home health-oncology services, client-managed obstetrical services, and same-day surgical services;
4. *Introduction of an innovation.* Examples of this include a new drug therapy, a computer system, outcome charting, and a complex instrument or machine (Drucker, 1974; Lewin, 1951).

Anyone who has been involved in health care QA activities will quickly recognize these categories as potential issues for a QA committee to address.

Because of his or her designated responsibilities, the QAC must understand the change process and anticipate the potential responses to it. The QAC also needs a repertoire of strategies that can facilitate the implementation of change since individuals are motivated by different forces.

CLASSIC CHANGE THEORIES

A number of theories has been developed to explain how change occurs. Some theorists have a behavioral or developmental view and perceive change as occurring primarily between and within individuals. Others have a system approach and view change as an interaction within a particular system and its subsystems. Another group combines the two approaches in describing the change process.

An overview of several classic change theories follows. Bear in mind that the sequential stages (phases or steps) identified in each theory are fluid and dynamic. In other words, the process can fluctuate between stages, move quickly from one to another, remain fixed at some point for long periods, or regress to a previous stage.

Due to space limitations and the fact that the stages in Lippitt's, Havelock's, and the eclectic theories are somewhat self-explanatory, these will not be elaborated on in detail. The reader who is interested in a particular theory is encouraged to review relevant works noted in the reference section.

Lewin's Force-Field Model (1951)

Classic change theory has its origins in the works of Kurt Lewin, who described change as progressing through three stages: (1) unfreezing, (2) moving, and (3) refreezing.

Unfreezing

In the stage of unfreezing, the motivation to create change occurs when there is a stressor, unrest, or conflict within a system. At other times, the motivation for change may arise from the realization that something can be done more easily or better. In general, the initial impetus for change arises when expectations are not being met (lack of confirmation), when discomfort exists about some action or lack of action (guilt and/or anxiety), or when an existing obstacle to change has been removed (threats to psychological well-being).

During this phase, the process is planned out in detail, and the system is readied for the change. This may include assessing the attitudes of those associates who work in a particular unit. This phase essentially means laying the preliminary groundwork for adoption of the change. For the QAC, this could be identifying a nursing problem on a particular unit or establishing a need for reorganizing a dysfunctional unit. Once the problem is identified, a study is undertaken to elicit relevant facts. For example, surveys may be needed to ascertain attitudes regarding the problem, or education may be necessary to promote awareness of the need for change.

Moving

The actual changing (moving) is Lewin's second stage. At this time, new responses (behaviors) are implemented based on the problem. Lewin encourages considering a problem from new perspectives (collecting data) via identification and/or scanning.

Identification occurs when a highly regarded peer, leader, or superior influences the change agent's decision about a potential resolution to solve a problem. This approach has the disadvantage of limiting awareness of alternative solutions. However, this mode might ensure the success of a planned change if the individual is viewed as a leader within the system.

Scanning, on the other hand, yields similar information about a problem, but data are collected from a variety of sources. The result is more options from which to choose. A disadvantage of this mode is that it can increase organizational decision-making time.

Restraining versus Driving Forces

Lewin believes that driving forces facilitate the implementation of change, while restraining forces impede it. For this reason, when planning change, a system assessment is needed to determine those factors that can be capitalized on and those that should be counterbalanced. It is important for a QAC to be aware that many carefully planned and much needed changes have failed to come to fruition because restraining and driving forces were not addressed.

Refreezing

Lewin's last stage, refreezing, occurs when a change or innovation is integrated into an organization's values. In other words, the changee assimilates the new behavior into existing practices and continues indefinitely without being reminded to do so.

For the QAC, this means following up on problems that have been investigated, particularly those implementing new practice protocols. This is particularly relevant in cases where a scientifically based practice is selected to replace well-established, (ritualistic) practice (e.g., intravenous site care, charting, or biomedical equipment maintenance).

Lippitt's Model (1973)

Lippitt focuses on problem solving and interpersonal dynamics having a major role in the change process. His theory is useful for the consultation process, another role that often is assumed by the QAC.

Exhibit 12-1 Lewin's and Lippitt's Theories of Change Compared

---

Unfreezing: (1) Diagnosing the problem

(2) Assessing the motivation and capacity for change

(3) Assessing the client's motivation and resources

Moving: (4) Selecting progressive objectives (strategies) for the change process

(5) Choosing and revising the roles used by the change agent

Refreezing: (6) Maintaining the change

(7) Terminating the change relationship

Source: From *Field Theory in Social Science* by K. Lewin, 1951, New York: Harper & Row, and from *Visualizing Change: Model Building and the Change Process* by G. Lippitt, 1973, LaJolla, CA: University Associates.

Exhibit 12-1 compares Lewin's model with Lippitt's seven-phase model. For the unfreezing phase, Lippit has three phases that focus on a careful assessment of the client system: determining the available resources, motivating change, and making an accurate diagnosis of the problem. His fourth stage (selecting appropriate change strategies) and fifth stage (choosing and revising the roles for the change agent) compare with Lewin's moving phase. Finally, Lippitt's last two stages—maintaining the change and terminating the change relationship—are incorporated in Lewin's refreezing phase.

Havelock's Model (1973)

Havelock's theory of change reflects the imporance of comprehensive preliminary data collecting and planning. The change agent's role is described by Havelock as active with a preference for the participative management approach. This means that staff nurses may initiate activities traditionally assumed by management. It also means that initial efforts in planning a change often require the greatest amount of time and resources. Nevertheless, significant changes, particularly in knowledge and attitudes, tend to occur during these preliminary activities. He divides the change process into six phases, as illustrated in Exhibit 12-2.

Havelock's stages of establishing rapport, diagnosing the problem, and acquiring the necessary resources to implement the change are comparable to Lewin's unfreezing stage. He expands on Lewin's moving phase with choosing an appropriate solution and gaining acceptance of the change. Finally, Havelock interprets refreezing to mean stabilizing the change and bringing about self-renewal within the system.

Exhibit 12-2 Lewin's and Havelock's Theories of Change Compared

Unfreezing: (1) Establishing rapport in the relationship
(2) Diagnosing the problem to implement appropriate change
(3) Acquiring the necessary resources to bring about the change
Moving: (4) Choosing an appropriate solution(s)
(5) Gaining acceptance of the change by the changee
Refreezing: (6) Stabilizing the change and bringing about self-renewal.

Source: From the *Change Agent's Guide to Innovation in Education* by R. Havelock, 1973, Englewood Cliffs, NJ: Educational Technology Publications, and from *Field Theory in Social Science* by K. Lewin, 1951, New York: Harper & Row.

Eclectic Model for Change versus the Nursing Process

As evidenced in the previous models, there are overlaps in the change processes and differences in terminology, as well as differing conceptual nuances among the theorists. The models do not focus on the specific vocabulary of nursing; thus, Sullivan and Decker (1988) provide an eclectic model for change that addresses the nursing process. Exhibit 12-3 compares the two.

As outlined in the exhibit, the nursing process consists of assessing, planning, implementing, and evaluating. The Eclectic Model of the change process consists of identifying the problem, collecting the data, analyzing the data, planning the change strategies, implementing the change, evaluating the effectiveness of the change, and stabilizing the change. In essence, the eclectic model is similar to

Exhibit 12-3 Seven Steps of Planned Change: An Extension of the Nursing Process

Nursing Process	Change Process
1. Assessing	1. Identifying the problem
	2. Collecting the data
	3. Analyzing the data
2. Planning	4. Planning the strategies
3. Implementing	5. Implementing the change
4. Evaluating	6. Evaluating the effectiveness
	7. Stabilizing the change

Source: From *Effective Management in Nursing*, 2nd ed., (p. 103) by E. Sullivan and P. Decker, 1988, Menlo Park, CA: Addison-Wesley Publishing Co. Copyright 1988 by Addison-Wesley Publishing Co. Reprinted by permission.

Lippitt's and Havelocks' in the up-front planning process, but it incorporates nursing language.

Rogers' Theory of Innovation and Diffusion of Change

Rogers' model focuses on the diffusion (dissemination) and adoption (acceptance) of innovations (Rogers, 1971; 1983; Rogers & Shoemaker, 1971). The model proposes that acceptance or rejection is determined by antecedents that influence the outcome. In other words, a person's experiences and values and the environment in which the change occurs motivate him or her to adopt or reject an innovation. Rogers delineates five phases in the diffusion process, elaborates on the adoption phase, and describes attributes that facilitate adoption/rejection of an innovation.

In essence, Exhibit 12-4 shows Rogers' perception of how an individual, or a group, passes from initial awareness of an innovation to acceptance or rejection of it. For instance, with quality assurance, through reading a professional journal a staff nurse *becomes aware of* an innovative flow sheet for monitoring intake and output (I & O) on burn patients. The nurse *evaluates* the appropriateness of the instrument for the burn unit of that hospital. Thereafter, the nurse and three peers agree to *try* the new instrument on a small scale in their unit and compare its outcomes with the existing methods of recording I & O. After the pilot test, the nurses recommend to their nursing manager and the QAC that the new flow sheet

---

Exhibit 12-4 Rogers' Theory of Diffusion and Adoption of Innovations

1. Awareness
2. Evaluation
3. Trial
4. Adoption (acceptance)
   a. Knowledge
   b. Persuasion
   c. Decision
   d. Implementation
5. Outcomes
   a. Accepted but change can be continued (integrated) or subsequently discontinued
   b. Rejected (not adopted), but change can either remain rejected or later be adopted in a modified form

Source: From *Social Change in Rural Society* by E. Rogers, 1971, Englewood Cliffs, NJ: Prentice-Hall, and from *Communication of Innovations: A Cross-Cultural Approach*, 1971, New York: Free Press.

be adopted on their unit. Their recommendation is based on its ease of use and degree of accuracy for reporting I & O on burn patients. In addition, the trial period allowed for modifications to be incorporated in the flow sheet. These minor revisions specifically addressed the idiosyncrasies of this particular burn unit.

Rogers' model also considers the reversible nature of change. For instance, a change may be adopted, but later it can be discontinued. Or the reverse—initially the change is rejected, but later it is adopted by the changee (Drucker, 1974, 1985a, 1985b; Rogers, 1971, 1983). The staff on the burn unit could experience either outcome in their use of the innovative I & O flow sheet.

Example Innovation: Electronic Thermometers

Consider the pattern of diffusion and adoption of a common innovation in health care, the electronic thermometer. When it was first developed about two decades ago, one read about the device in science journals. Several years later, these thermometers were described in the more widely read nursing journals, and recently in popular women's magazines.

After the model was first developed, research medical centers purchased the costly item for a few specialty units. The primary use of the thermometer was to determine its accuracy in recording temperatures and its cost effectiveness as determined by time-motion studies. After the innovation became available (diffused) at the local level by pharmaceutical supply companies and medical equipment houses, additional hospitals purchased the innovation. It was beginning to be an "established standard of practice."

A few years later, electronic thermometers were mass produced, the instruments had additional capabilities due to the introduction of computer chip technology, and their price was greatly reduced. Then a media blitz was undertaken by manufacturers in order to inform consumers, nurses in particular, of their cost effectiveness, safety features, and accuracy in monitoring patients. As a result of these efforts, most hospitals purchased one for each clinical unit. More than two decades after the invention of the thermometer, one can purchase them in a wide variety of retail stores.

Use (adoption) of the thermometers by nurses is also typical of other innovations. Initially, most "tried out the novelty." After a period of time, some used it "only when the supervisor was in the area." A few stated that they never used it and that it merely sits on the desk. At the other end of the spectrum, a few adopters state they "can't provide quality patient care without an electronic thermometer." After almost three decades, resisters state that because electronic thermometers are inaccurate and never work when they need them, they prefer to use the standard thermometer.

Recently, another innovation intended to address the serious health risk of AIDS and other infectious diseases has been introduced and broadly disseminated:

universal isolation precautions. Consequently, infrequent users (nonadopters) are finding the thermometer a requirement to implement these protocols. The reliability of the thermometer has been improved because of the availability of cellular, self-charging batteries.

For the QAC, the adoption pattern of the electronic thermometer can provide useful insights. In cases where a change is initially rejected, one shoud not assume an issue is dead. Sometimes a change can be resurrected, perhaps in an altered form or at a more opportune time when external and internal forces facilitate the process. Likewise, if a change is accepted, one cannot assume permanence by those who have initially accepted.

Adoption

Rogers elaborates on phases in the adoption process. In the knowledge stage, an individual is exposed to the innovation, begins to understand how it functions, and identifies the benefits/risks for those who use it. The persuasion stage is a period during which attitudes are formed about the innovation via the acquisition of pertinent information. The decision stage is a period during which information about the innovation is evaluated and analyzed, which may result in trial use of it. At this time, the innovation is accepted or rejected.

During the implementation stage, the innovation is utilized on a more permanent basis. The organization may restructure itself to accommodate the innovation—or the innovation may be modified to "fit" within the organization.

The final stage, confirmation, occurs when individuals seek reinforcement of their decision to either adopt or reject the innovation. If conflicting messages are experienced by the system, or if the costs seem to outweight the benefits, the decision may be reversed.

Rogers lists antecedents that influence adoption. These complement and enhance Lewin's concept of driving and restraining forces and are termed as relative advantage, compatibility, complexity, trialability, or divisibility, and communicability.

Relative advantage is the degree to which an organization perceives the innovation as making things better or easier for those who adopt it. It is not important whether or not there is an actual improvement. Rather, the important facet is that which the client *perceives or believes* to be a benefit or a disadvantage of the innovation.

Compatibility refers to the degree of similarity between an innovation and an organization's existing value system. For QA changes, this refers to an institution's mission, philosophy, practice norms, organizational structure, and internal/external regulatory mandates, as well as its views of formal and informal leaders.

Complexity refers to the innovation's degree of sophistication, particularly its mechanical complexity (or simplicity). In general, unfamiliar skills or those that are difficult for a user to develop result in rejection of the innovation, while those innovations that require less complicated techniques seem to be adopted more readily. Likewise, changes that are more concrete in nature (e.g., newly designated parking areas, use of time-clocks by employees) are easier to get accepted than are those that are more abstract in nature (e.g., use of computers, quality assurance). This may be related to the fact that the latter often have an esoteric vocabulary, making them less easily understood.

Once understood and accepted, complex innovations tend to persist, whereas less complex ones do not. This may result because a simple innovation does not have sufficient complexity to survive modifications that must be made when adopted at various hierarchical levels. A simple innovation tends to be lost or modified to such an extent that it no longer can be recognized in its original form.

Trialability refers to the degree to which an innovation is divisible—that is, the ease with which it can be implemented on a small scale or in a pilot study. The more prevalent this attribute is, the greater the chance for adoption is. Small-scale trials provide an opportunity to solve previously unanticipated problems and to influence resisters' attitudes, thereby facilitating large-scale adoption.

Communicability refers to the ease with which the innovation can be described. The easier it is to explain, the more likely it is to be accepted, which may be related to the complexity of thought needed to grasp an innovation (e.g., abstract versus concrete concepts, familiar versus unfamiliar vocabularies).

Selection of Change Strategies

An innovation's attributes, as well as the point at which the changee is in the adoption process, influence the strategies a QAC selects to implement a change (Lancaster & Lancaster, 1982; Stevens, 1975; Vroom, 1964; Ward & Moran, 1984; Welsh, 1979). For instance, during the awareness stage, mass media techniques (such as pamphlets, radio broadcasts, news letters, and/or fact sheets) may be most effective.

The information, as well as the method in which it is disseminated (e.g., professional literature, research utilization committees, journal club, or literature that depicts a "task analysis" of the innovation) may change during the persuasion stage. Strategies that are more effective during the decision stage (which leads into the evaluation stage) include scheduling educational inservice classes, providing practice sessions, and implementing small-scale use of the innovation.

To be effective, all of these activities should be followed by a debriefing session to elicit feelings, ideas, and attitudes from attendants. Discussions of this type provide an opportunity to expose associates to peers' and supervisors' views and promote feelings of ownership among associates. Debriefing also encourages a thorough analysis and provides an opportunity to make modifications in the change that facilitate an organizational fit (Haffer, 1986; Hickman & Silva, 1984; Rowland & Rowland, 1980).

Once a change is implemented, face-to-face communication may be the most effective means of maintaining it. Nonetheless, a QAC still must focus on modifying the innovation as the need arises. If rejected, efforts should be undertaken to determine restraining or impeding factors. Sometimes the problem may need to be redefined in light of new information, and this may require reformulation of solutions. For those who resist, another innovation may be needed, as in the case of electronic thermometers. To reiterate, not all change is successfully implemented because the complexity of the process and the wide range of human responses to change intervene.

APPLICATION OF LEWIN'S PRINCIPLES OF CHANGE

Several principles have been found to be relevant to all change (Lewin, 1951), and these are useful also for QA activities.

1. *There is an almost universal tendency to seek to maintain the status quo on the part of those whose needs are being met.* Or, to rephrase, when things are going well, most individuals see no need for change, nor are they likely to accept change during these times (Rogers, 1971).

2. *Resistance to change increases in direct proportion to the degree to which change is perceived as a threat.* The more an individual has to lose, the more intense the feelings of resistance are. Conversely, the more the change is congruent with existing values and the perceived personal benefits, the more likely it is to be accepted. From this premise evolves the change strategy of providing information about the change that has meaning on a personal level (Drucker 1985a, 1985b; Stevens, 1975).

3. *Resistance to change increases in direct response to pressure to change.* Prochange forces within an organization rock the boat, alter the status quo, and motivate change. These forces may surface in the form of organizational pain, discomfort, inefficient functioning, inability to meet goals, and/or ineffective interpersonal interactions. Antichange forces, on the other hand, work toward maintaining the equilibrium, but despite pain or dysfunction, there remains a reward of some sort for resisters (Quinn, 1985; Rogers, 1971).

For instance, the QAC may find that a nursing unit avoids reorganizing staffing patterns despite increased patient acuity profiles. By continuing with existing practices, the staff can remain in familiar (nonthreatening) patterns of interaction with supervisors, peers, and patients, even though the unit is not cost effective.

4. *Resistance to change decreases when it is perceived as being reinforced by trusted others, such as high-prestige figures, those whose judgment is respected, and those of like mind.* Two highly influential components of successful change

are (1) that key leaders within an organization are interested in the innovation and (2) that these individuals are committed to making it happen (Drucker, 1974, 1985a, 1985b; Rogers, 1983).

Thus, a useful change strategy for a QAC is to seek support from the formal leaders (administration), as well as the informal leaders, in an organization. This means encouraging managers to attend unit/department QA meetings, requesting that management directives demonstrate support for quality assurance, and publishing "News Notes of QA" to recognize active associates, who often tend to be the informal leaders (Katz & Kahn, 1978; Rogers, 1971, 1983).

5. *Resistance to change decreases when those involved are able to foresee how they might establish a new equilibrium that is as good or better than the old.* Knowledge about the risks and benefits of an innovation can facilitate adoption. For instance, sharing firsthand experiences via word of mouth is a useful strategy when replacing well-established behaviors (e.g., poor practice, ritualistic interventions) with an innovation that has as its goal improved practice (e.g., research-based nursing intervention, use of sophisticated biomedical equipment) (Brucks, 1985; Drucker, 1985a, 1985b). Other strategies include providing formal and informal educational opportunities, viewing audiovisual materials (often provided by manufacturers), participating in professional conferences, and making professional reading materials accessible on a nursing unit.

Generally, those who read about an innovation in professional journals are more likely to adopt it, as compared to those who do not read. Thus, organizing a unit-specific journal club that focuses on relevant QA reports and encouraging "use of a library time" are two strategies that promote professional awareness and also enhance peer support (Chinn, 1969; del Bueno, 1985).

From this discussion, it becomes obvious that the setting (corporate culture) impacts on acceptance of change. An organization's infrastructure can deter or facilitate adoption of change (e.g., centralized versus decentralized management). Likewise, failure to accept a change that results from QA findings may be associated with the cost (time, energy, personnel, resources), the extent and mode of dissemination, the degree of perceived administrative support, and the amount of perceived ownership by associates. External regulatory agencies (e.g., Joint Commission on Accreditation of Healthcare Organizations, state health department, Medicare) also can influence adoption. Another institutional determinant is educational level of the associates, particularly of midlevel managers and those who are actively involved in implementing the change. Whether these individuals are not informed about or committed to the idea, inadvertently or perhaps advertently, will be reflected in their day-to-day interactions.

6. *Commitment to change increases when those involved have the opportunity to participate in the decisions to make and to implement the change.* Individuals are more apt to adopt an idea if they have ownership. For this reason, the QAC should encourage active participation by all who are impacted by the change. Discussion is needed to facilitate awareness, foster critical analysis, and develop

modifications to ensure that the innovation is congruent with the organizations's values (Porter & Lawler, 1968; Rogers, 1971; Stevens, 1975).

To encourage support and involvement, associates should be notified of and involved in a proposed change prior to its implementation. Through a participative management style, a QAC will find that professionals can provide valuable insights as to the actual problem, identify potential solutions, anticipate the ramifications of each, and initiate a change that fits with the hospital's objectives and goals. This can be accomplished through verbal and/or written announcement(s).

A guiding principle in participative management is to disseminate at least three general announcements at various times before implementing a change. Depending on the magnitude of the change, the announcements can be made years, months, weeks, or days in advance. As the time draws near to implement the change, keep associates actively involved in the process, apprise them of any expectations, and inform them of anticipated outcomes (Pincus, 1986; Rogers 1971, 1983).

The QAC must be sensitive to timing issues. For example, when several planned changes are being considered, they must be prioritized in accordance with long-range goals. Introducing several changes at once can "overload" a system. For this reason, time must be built in for each change to be integrated into existing behaviors (American Nurses' Association, 1980; Beer, 1981; Drucker, 1985a, 1985b; Fickeissen, 1985; Ganong & Ganong, 1983; Geolot, 1986; Green, 1983; Ignatavicius, 1983; Schwirian, 1978, 1981; Stevens, 1975).

7. *Resistance to change is based on fear of the new circumstances. Fear is decreased when those involved have the opoportunity to experience these new circumstances under conditions of minimal threat.* As discussed previously, trials facilitate modifications that promote organization-innovation congruency.

8. *Temporary alterations in most situations can be brought about by the use of direct pressure, such as an administrative directive; however, this activity is accompanied by heightened tension, which will yield a highly unstable situation.* The coercive-power approach was highly evident when quality assurance was initially mandated by external regulatory agencies. This strategy is quick, and apparently effective, to resolve an immediate problem. In the long run, though, this may not be the most effective means to bring about a permanent change. Administrative directives tend to create distrust, lower morale, and promote passive-aggressive responses among subordinates. In part, this is due to the lack of a sense of ownership by subordinates, as evidenced by reduced productivity, lowered quality of work, wasted time, and antagonistic attitudes directed toward supervisors (Kjervik, 1984; Rogers, 1983).

CONCLUSION

Change does not occur in a vacuum. Moreover, the QAC, as well as non-manager staff nurses, must recognize that all changes have benefits and costs.

Whether a change is adopted or rejected by associates will depend on the accurate identification of the problem, the selection of the most appropriate solution, the involvement of associates, and the skills of the change agent, as well as the environment in which the change is implemented.

REFERENCES

American Nurses Association. (1980). *Nursing: A social policy statement*. Kansas City, MO: Author.

Beer, M. (1981). Performance appraisal: Dilemmas and possibilities. *Organizational Dynamics*, (Spring), 24.

Bennis, W., Benne, K., & Chinn, R. (1969). *The planning of change* (2nd ed.). New York: Holt, Rinehart & Winston.

Boncarosky, L.D. (1979). Guidelines to corrective discipline. *Personnel Journal* (October), 698.

Brooten, D., Hayman, L., & Naylor, M. (1988). *Leadership for change: An action guide for nurses*. Philadelphia: J.B. Lippincott.

Brucks, A. (1985). Performance appraisal: Evaluating the evaluation. *The Healthcare Supervisor*, *3*(4), 17–30.

Chinn, R. (1969). The utility of systems models and developmental models for practitioners. In W. Bennis, K. Benne, & R. Chinn (Eds.), *The planning of change* (2nd ed.) (pp. 297–312). New York: Holt, Rinehart & Winston.

del Bueno, D.J. (1985). Bandwagons, parades and pancreas. *Nursing Outlook, 33*(3), 136–138.

Drucker, P. (1974). *Management: Tasks, responsibilities, practice*. New York: Harper & Row.

Drucker, P. (1985a). The discipline of innovation. *Harvard Business Review, 63*(3), 67–72.

Drucker, P. (1985b). *Innovations and entrepreneurship*. New York: Harper & Row.

Fickeissen, J. (1985). Getting certified. *American Journal of Nursing, 85*(3), 265–269.

Ganong, J., & Ganong, W. (1983). *Performance appraisal for productivity: The nurse manager's handbook*. Gaithersburg, MD: Aspen Publishers.

Geolot, P. (1986). The relationship between certification and practice. *Nurse Practitioner, 11*(3), 55–58.

Green, C. (1983). Teaching strategies for the process of planned change. *Journal of Continuing Education in Nursing, 14*(6), 16–23.

Haffer, A. (1986). Facilitating change: Choosing the appropriate strategy. *Journal of Nursing Administration, 16*(4), 18–22.

Havelock, R. (1973). *The change agent's guide to innovation in education*. New Jersey: Educational Technology Publications.

Havelock, R., & Havelock, M. (1973). *Training for change agents*. Ann Arbor, MI: University of Michigan Press.

Hersey, P., & Blanchard, K. (1977). *Management of organizational behavior*. Englewood Cliffs, NJ: Prentice-Hall.

Hickman, C., & Silva, M. (1984). *Creating excellence: Managing corporate culture, strategy and change in the new age*. New York: New American Library.

Ignatavicius, D. (1983). Clinical competence of new graduates: A study to measure performance. *Journal of Continuing Education in Nursing, 14*(4), 17–20.

Katz D., & Kahn, R. (1978). *The social psychology of organizations* (2nd ed.). New York: Wiley.

Kjervik, D. (1984). Progressive discipline in nursing: Arbitrators' decisions. *Journal of Nursing Administration, 14*(4), 34.

Lachman, V. (1984). Increasing productivity through performance evaluation. *Journal of Nursing Administration, 14*(12), 7–14.

Lancaster, J., & Lancaster, W. (1982). *The nurse as change agent.* St. Louis: C.V. Mosby.

Lewin, K. (1951). *Field theory in social science.* New York: Harper & Row.

Lippitt, G. (1973). *Visualizing change: Model building and the change process.* LaJolla, CA: University Associates.

Lippitt, R., Watson, J., & Westley, B. (1958). *The dynamics of planned change.* New York: Harcourt, Brace.

McCloskey, J. (1983a). Nursing education and job effectiveness. *Nursing Research, 32*(2), 53–58.

McCloskey, J. (1983b). *Toward an educational model of nursing effectiveness.* Ann Arbor, MI: UMI Research Press.

McCloskey, J., & McCain, B. (1987). Satisfaction, commitment and professionalism of newly employed nurses. *IMAGE: Journal of Nursing Scholarship, 19*(1), 20–24.

Marriner, A. (1979). Planned change as a leadership strategy. *Nursing Leadership, 2*(2), 11–14.

Naisbitt, J. (1983). *Megatrends.* New York: Warner Books.

Peplau, H. (1987). Is nursing's self-regulatory power being eroded? *Journal of the New York State Nurses' Association, 18*(3), 13–17.

Peters, T., & Austin, N. (1985). *A passion for excellence.* New York: Warner Books.

Pincus, J. (1986). Communication: Key contributor to effectiveness—The research. *Journal of Nursing Administration, 16*(9), 19–25.

Porter, L., & Lawler, E. (1968). *Managerial attitudes and performance.* Homewood, IL: Irwin & Dorsey Press.

Price, J., & Mueller, C. (1981). *Professional turnover: The case of the nurses.* New York: Spectrum.

Quinn, J. (1985). Managing innovation: Controlled chaos. *Harvard Business Review, 72*(3), 73–84.

Rakich, J., Longest, B., & O'Donovan, T. (1977). *Managing health care organizations.* Philadelphia: Saunders.

Rogers, E. (1971). *Social change in rural society.* Englewood Cliffs, NJ: Prentice-Hall.

Rogers, E. (1983). *Diffusion of innovations* (3rd ed.). New York: Free Press.

Rogers, E., & Shoemaker, F. (1971). *Communication of innovations: A cross-cultural approach.* New York: Free Press.

Rowland, H., & Rowland, B. (1980). *Nursing administration handbook.* Gaithersburg, MD: Aspen Publishers.

Schwirian, P. (1978). Evaluating the performance of nurses: A multidimensional approach. *Nursing Research, 27*(6), 347–351.

Schwirian, P. (1981). Toward an explanatory model of nursing performance. *Nursing Research, 30*(4), 247–253.

Stevens, B. (1975). Effecting change. *Journal of Nursing Administration, 5*(4), 23–26.

Stull, M. (1986). Staff nurse performance: Effects of goal-setting and performance feedback. *Journal of Nursing Administration, 16*(7, 8), 26–30.

Sullivan, E., & Decker, P. (1988). *Effective management in nursing.* Menlo Park, CA.: Addison-Wesley.

Toffler, A. (1970). *Future Shock.* New York: Bantam Books.

Vroom, V. (1964). *Work and motivation*. Malabar, FL: Robert E. Krieger.

Ward, M., & Moran, S. (1984). Resistance to change: Reorganize, respond, overcome. *Nursing Management, 15*(1), 30–33.

Welsh, L. (1979). Planned change in nursing: The theory. *Nursing Clinics of North America, 14*(2), 307–321.

13

Monitoring and Evaluation: Conclusions and Directions

Patricia Schroeder, MSN, RN, Quality Care Consultant, Quality Care Concepts, Thiensville, Wisconsin

At first glance, the process of monitoring and evaluation described in this book appears concrete and straightforward. One must collect data and take action based on the results. Those of us who have actually used this approach to improve care understand that the process is inherently more complex.

Monitoring and evaluating for quality forces participants to make statements about their beliefs. The clinical issues about which we collect data are selected based on the belief that they have an important clinical impact and are patient outcomes sensitive to professional nursing practice. The way the data are used speaks to the degree to which those involved feel empowered to create change within the organization. Finally, organizational values are identified by virtue of who has been accountable to make decisions about what to monitor and how to improve. The monitoring and evaluation program in a clinical agency says a great deal about the values held.

The preceding chapters demonstrate growth in the conduct of monitoring and evaluation activities. Whereas not long ago, nurses struggled with where to start, today we work on refinements in systems. Nurses began monitoring practice by collecting data on anything that seemed quantifiable. We have since evolved and ask new questions related to identification of those measures that accurately reflect the impact of professional nursing on patient outcomes. But while strides have been made, struggles continue; and while differences among specialty practice areas are present, some dilemmas are common.

Nurses in all settings continue to work to create efficient approaches to integrating established standards of practice and care with monitoring and evaluation activities. Today's outcome-oriented health care climate pushes us beyond an analysis of the how-tos of nursing practice and documentation and requires us to look at the ultimate impact of care on patient well-being. Multidisciplinary quality assurance (QA) activities are increasingly necessary because of the collaborative impact of interventions and require different skills, systems, and relationships.

271

Programs for monitoring and evaluation also present continuing dilemmas. Nurses continue to work at building monitoring and evaluation activities into the roles of all practitioners. This approach is supported by quality improvement philosophies used successfully outside of the health care industry. Such philosophies build the measurement of quality into every worker's role.

The automation of quality data is in its infancy, but will provide great assistance and raise further questions for quality assurance. Nurses will need to further develop their skills in creating data sets, integrating variables, and using large data bases. Given the rapid advancement of computer technology, it is interesting to note how little advancement has been made in actual approaches to QA applications and data management. As the importance of quality is recognized, and as identification of essential clinical indicators is refined, technology will be increasingly available and used for quality assurance.

The evolution of monitoring and evaluation will not, however, be limited to influences within the clinical agency. Quality indicators are and will increasingly be measured by or for federal and state agencies, accrediting bodies, third-party payers, professional review organizations, and consumers. Sophisticated automation will be required to integrate quality data with issues of cost, productivity, and access. The large data bases necessary to contain these data must be developed and used astutely. It is critical to assure that the importance of nursing in achieving quality patient outcomes is visible throughout. Nurses must play a role in creating the future, rather than merely reacting to it.

Nurses, patients, and others can cite innumerable examples of how quality nursing care was the determining factor in achieving positive patient outcomes. Conversely, we have all heard about those patients who have had accurate medical diagnoses and treatment, yet faired poorly due to inadequate nursing care. Some clinical indicator sets, developed to reflect quality patient care and currently being tested for national use, predominantly identify indicators of medical practice. Positive patient outcomes are most likely to be achieved through the organized collaboration of knowledgeable, skilled, and compassionate health care professionals. As we seek to measure and improve the quality of care, clinical indicators must also accurately reflect the true scope of care received. Any indicator set, national or otherwise, that does not do so misrepresents the health care system, is destructive to those practitioners not identified, and ultimately does a disservice to the well-being of the American public.

As the use of specific quality indicators becomes increasingly mandated, the profession of nursing must speak with a united voice and assure the inclusion of nurse-sensitive patient outcomes in the indicator sets. Nurses in clinical agencies must continue to identify, measure, and analyze quality indicators that speak to the clinical outcomes achieved by their patients. We must use these data to improve patient care. And we must then share the indicators to increase our impact on patient well-being, as well as to attempt to gain greater consensus on appropriate indicators for use.

Ultimately, the value of monitoring and evaluation is not in the creation of data or reports, but in the use of such data to improve care. Patients and families must be better off for such programs, or we have failed. Monitoring and evaluation continue to evolve and expand on organizational, corporate, and national levels. They can only make an impact, however, if they accurately reflect that which occurs at the bedside.

Index

275

N